VIRTUAL
EXERCISE PHYSIOLOGY
LABORATORY

CD-ROM With Lab Manual

VIRTUAL EXERCISE PHYSIOLOGY LABORATORY

CD-ROM With Lab Manual

Fred W. Kolkhorst, PhD, FACSM
Michael J. Buono, PhD, FACSM

San Diego State University

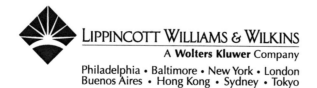

LIPPINCOTT WILLIAMS & WILKINS
A **Wolters Kluwer** Company

Philadelphia • Baltimore • New York • London
Buenos Aires • Hong Kong • Sydney • Tokyo

Editor: Peter Darcy
Development Editor: David Payne
Marketing Manager: Christen DeMarco
Project Editor: Jennifer D.W. Glazer
Designer: Doug Smock
Compositor: LWW
Printer: Victor Graphics

351 West Camden Street
Baltimore, Maryland 21201

530 Walnut Street
Philadelphia, Pennsylvania 19106

Library of Congress Cataloging-in-Publication has been applied for.
ISBN-13: 978-0-7817-3608-4
ISBN-10: 0-7817-3608-0

To purchase additional copies of this book, call our customer service department at **(800) 638-3030** or fax orders to **(301) 824-7390**. For other book services, including chapter reprints and large quantity sales, ask for the Special Sales department.

For all other calls originating outside of the United States, please call **(301)714-2324.**

Visit Lippincott Williams & Wilkins on the Internet: http://www.lww.com. Lippincott Williams & Wilkins customer service representatives are available from 8:30 am to 6:00 pm, EST, Monday through Friday, for telephone access.

PREFACE

The emphasis of the *Virtual Exercise Physiology Laboratory* is on developing student understanding, rather than the collecting and recognizing descriptive data, by connecting the physiology to observations during an exercise test. Instructors and students can be assured that data collected in a virtual investigation will fall within an expected response. In addition, physiological variables not normally measured in an undergraduate or even graduate exercise physiology laboratory can be obtained in a virtual investigation. Plasma catecholamine concentrations, muscle, skin, and splanchnic blood flows, and muscle glycogen levels are but a few of the measures possible during a virtual experiment. The learning benefit of these measures is to assist student understanding of the physiological mechanisms that explain metabolic and hemodynamic responses to exercise. Training studies, which cannot be conducted in a semester course, can be quickly performed to demonstrate metabolic and cardiovascular adaptations to regular exercise. Moreover, altitude studies are available to show the metabolic and cardiovascular responses to exercise in a hypoxic environment; thermoregulation studies can be performed to demonstrate the effects of heat stress, the benefits of maintaining fluid balance and adaptation to exercise in the heat; and aging and gender effects on exercise can be conducted.

Besides offering a variety of virtual activities, many of the standard exercise physiology laboratory experiments are included in this accompanying manual. This allows flexibility for instructors to choose those activities that he/she feels best fits the needs of the course and students. The laboratory activities are grouped as:

- *Demonstration*—Instructor demonstration of an important exercise physiology test, e.g., $\dot{V}O_{2max}$ test.

- *Student activity investigation*—Individual or small-group investigations in which all students are actively involved in data collection, e.g., HR and BP responses to exercise.

- *Virtual investigation*—Independent study using the *Virtual Exercise Physiology Laboratory* to investigate the mechanisms that explain a physiological response to exercise.

- *Student inquiry investigation*—Small-group investigation in which fewer guidelines are provided. Students are required to take a more active role in designing and conducting the experiment.

The variety of activities included in the manual allows the instructor to preserve standard activities that fit his/her course philosophies and laboratory capabilities, as well as including ones that previously could not be covered because of equipment limitations. For instance, the instructor could choose to demonstrate a lactate threshold test to students, and then assign students to conduct a similar virtual experiment. In this manner, the virtual investigation of changes in blood pH and plasma catecholamine concentrations helps students to understand occurrence of the ventilatory threshold and a primary reason for increased carbohydrate metabolism. Virtual investigations allow students, in either in- or out-of-class assignments, to conduct an experiment and obtain reasonable data from a wide range of physiologic and metabolic variables. Furthermore, students can manipulate a testing condition (e.g., training status, heat, altitude) and repeat the test on the same virtual subject to compare responses from a control trial. In addition, students and instructors can develop their own lab investigations on a variety of topics. The Box below lists the physiological measurements that can be used for virtual investigations.

Physiological Measurements Available on the Virtual Exercise Physiology Laboratory.

Cardiovascular Measures

cardiac output
heart rate
stroke volume
systolic blood pressure
diastolic blood pressure
mean arterial pressure
total peripheral resistance
rate-pressure product
muscle blood flow
splanchnic blood flow
capillary-to-fiber ratio
mixed a-v O_2 difference

Thermoregulation

core temperature
skin temperature
sweat rate
skin blood flow
hematocrit
plasma volume

Pulmonary Measures

oxygen uptake
carbon dioxide production
respiratory exchange ratio
minute ventilation
O_2 ventilatory equivalent
CO_2 ventilatory equivalent

Blood Glucose Regulation

blood glucose
insulin
glucagon
liver glucose output
liver glycogen
muscle glucose uptake

Sarcoplasmic Measures

ATP
PCr
muscle glycogen
mitochondria (% muscle cell)
% of ST fibers

Blood Measures

lactate
free fatty acids
free fatty acid uptake
glycerol
ketone bodies
epinephrine
norepinephrine
pH
bicarbonate

Muscle Enzymes

creatine kinase
myokinase
phosphorylase
phosphofructokinase
lactate dehydrogenase
succinate dehydrogenase
malate dehydrogenase
carnitine palmityl transferase
rating of perceived exertion

At the end of each laboratory experiment is a series of questions designed to lead a student to understand the reasoning for the responses observed in the experiment. Rather than stressing methodology or laboratory techniques, the learning emphasis is on the involved physiology. Many questions build on previous ones and connect different physiological systems to help the student understand how they interact during exercise.

The *Virtual Exercise Physiology Laboratory* was not designed to replace actual laboratory experiences. To be sure, the greatest potential for learning is for students to design an experiment to answer their own research question, conduct the experiment, and to analyze and present the results. Given the limitations of providing for an ideal laboratory experience, however, integrating the *Virtual Exercise Physiology Laboratory* into a laboratory course can overcome many of these limitations and permit learning experiences not possible in undergraduate, and most graduate, teaching laboratories.

INSTRUCTIONS FOR USING THE *VIRTUAL EXERCISE PHYSIOLOGY LABORATORY*

Using the *Virtual Exercise Physiology Laboratory* is simple! After the software loads, a window rises from the bottom of the screen prompting the user to select a subject to test and the parameters to measure. Under the **1) Select Subject & Test Condition** section, click on the desired test (Prolonged Time Trials or Incremental Speed Trials) and then on the desired subject within that test *(all clicks should be made with the left button on the mouse)*, which opens a pull-down menu listing the different testing conditions available for that subject. Choose the condition to be tested. Next, under the **2) Select Measurements** section, click on the category parameters to be measured and then click all the specific parameters. A yellow bullet will indicate the selected parameters. When ready to begin a test, click on the **OK** button.

To start a test, click on the **Resting Data** button, then on the **Start** button when ready to begin testing. The running test time is indicated in minutes and the treadmill speed is indicated in units of meters per minute. The program will prompt you when to take readings, but parameters will not be measured until you click on the **Take Readings** button. The test will continue until you click the **Stop** button or when the subject reaches exhaustion. While a test is being conducted, you can view the data in either the table format or graph format. To enlarge a graph for better viewing, click on the **Zoom** button; click on the **Close** button to reduce it back to its original size.

If, after completing a test, you want to perform another one, click on the **Setup** button, which will bring up the setup window. Click on the **Clear** button if you are performing a different protocol and do not wish to compare data from the second test to that from the first. There will be occasions, however, when you will want to compare data between different testing conditions or subjects. For example, you may want to compare the effects of training adaptation on cardiovascular parameters by testing an untrained subject and then testing her again after she has been training. Or, you may want to compare the effects of exercising at sea level with that at altitude. For these situations, don't clear the data in the graph memory. Rather, deselect the last test by clicking on it and then clicking on the new subject or testing condition. Data collected on subsequent tests will be laid over the graphs so that you can quickly compare responses between subjects or conditions.

CONTENTS

UNIT IV SPECIAL TOPICS 75

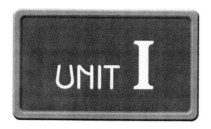

Introduction

UNITS OF MEASURE

Most measurements in science are reported using metric units, which are based on units that vary by powers of 10. Table 1 describes the commonly used prefixes and symbols.

To promote consistency in communication, most professional organizations, including the American College of Sports Medicine (ACSM), have adopted use of the Système International d'Unités (SI units)(Table 2). Use the following information to convert English and metric units to SI units. Proper expressions of the abbreviations are indicated in parentheses. Note that abbreviations of plural units are never followed with an "s," nor are they followed by a period. Abbreviations of units of measure are to be separated by a space from the number, and with few exceptions, the abbreviations are expressed in lowercase letters. Notable exceptions are the liter (L), Newton (N), Watt (W), and Joule (J). In addition, units expressed in exponential form are preferable to the use of a solidus (/) (e.g., $m \cdot s^{-1}$ instead of m/s; $mL \cdot kg^{-1} \cdot min^{-1}$ instead of mL/kg/min).

TABLE 1
Prefixes and symbols for metric units of length.

Prefix	Multiple	Symbol
nano	0.000000001 (10^{-9})	n
micro	0.000001 (10^{-6})	μ
milli	0.001 (10^{-3})	m
centi	0.01 (10^{-2})	c
deci	0.1 (10^{-1})	d
kilo	1000 (10^{3})	k
mega	1,000,000 (10^{6})	M
giga	1,000,000,000 (10^{9})	G

LENGTH

TABLE 2
Metric measures of length and conversion factors.

SI unit	Equivalent metric units	Equivalent English units
meter (m)	100 centimeters (cm)	1.093613 yards (yd)
	1000 millimeters (mm)	3.28084 feet (ft)
	1,000,000 micrometers (µm)	39.37008 inches (in)

To convert:	Multiply by:
feet to meters	0.304780
inches to meters	0.025380
meters to feet	3.28084
meters to inches	39.37008

MASS (WEIGHT)

Although these terms are often used interchangeably, they are actually different. Mass is an inherent property of a body that gives it inertia to resist changes in motion. Weight, on the other hand, is the force of gravity acting on the body (i.e., gravity × mass) and technically is a measure of force. To illustrate the difference between weight and mass, one's weight would be considerably less on the moon than on earth because the force of gravity is much less on the moon. However, body mass would be identical at the two locations. The English unit of weight is the pound and its metric equivalent is technically the Newton (N) rather than the kilogram (kg). Regardless, weight is traditionally expressed in the metric system with the unit being the kilogram (Table 3).

VOLUME

Volumes are greatly influenced by pressure and temperature, particularly gas volumes. To illustrate this point, although the number of gas molecules in a balloon measured at sea level and at altitude does not change, the balloon occupies a much greater volume at altitude. This demonstrates Boyle's Law, which states

TABLE 3
Metric units of mass and conversion factors.

SI unit	Equivalent metric units	Equivalent English units
kilogram (kg)	1000 grams (g)	2.204624 pounds (lb)

To convert:	Multiply by:
pounds to kilograms	0.453592
kilograms to pounds	2.204624

that volume is inversely proportional to pressure. Likewise, according to Charles' Law, which states that volume is directly proportional to pressure, the balloon volume would be greater in a hot environment than a cool one. Thus, in order to report gas volumes measured under different conditions, they must be mathematically corrected to represent the volume under a standardized condition. Typically, the rates of oxygen utilization and carbon dioxide production ($\dot{V}O_2$ and $\dot{V}CO_2$, respectively) are corrected to Standard Temperature, Pressure, and Dry (STPD) conditions. This indicates that the volume has been corrected to represent the gas volume if the temperature was 0 °C (273 °K), there was 1 atmosphere of pressure, and there was no water vapor in the gas. Lung capacities and volumes, though, are commonly expressed as Body Temperature, ambient Pressure, and Saturated (BTPS). In this case, the volume has been corrected to represent the gas at body temperature (37 °C or 310 °K), ambient pressure, and saturated with water vapor (which exerts a partial pressure of 47 mm Hg at 37 °C). However, when lung volumes and capacities are measured in the laboratory, they are done so under Ambient Temperature and Pressure, and Saturated with water vapor (ATPS). To convert an ATPS volume to BTPS, multiply the ATPS volume by the correction factor based on the ambient temperature (see Appendix P).

Although computerized metabolic measurement systems correct gas volumes in the computations, volumes measured by spirometers, and when expired gases are collected in Douglas bags or in meteorological balloons, must be subsequently corrected. Use the STPD correction factors found in Appendix O to correct expired air volumes for temperature and barometric pressure.

TEMPERATURE

- To convert Fahrenheit to Celsius: $°C = (°F - 32) \div 1.8$
- To convert Celsius to Fahrenheit: $°F = (1.8 \times °C) + 32$

SPEED (VELOCITY)

Although commonly used interchangeably, speed is the magnitude of velocity, while the accurate expression of velocity includes the direction of the movement as well as its magnitude. Speed is the rate at which something moves; thus, speed is expressed as the distance traveled divided by a unit of time (e.g., miles $\cdot$ h^{-1}) (Table 4).

FORCE

Force is defined as that which is applied to a body that causes it to move or to speed up (Table 5).

POWER AND WORK

Work is accomplished when a force acts on a body that causes it to move in the same direction; thus work is the product of force on the body and the distance

TABLE 4
Metric units of speed (velocity) and conversion factors.

SI unit	Equivalent metric units	Equivalent English units
meters per second (m · s^{-1})	3.6 kilometers per hour (km · h^{-1}) 0.0166667 meters per minute (m · min^{-1})	2.236936 miles per hour (miles · h^{-1})

To convert:	Multiply by:
meters per second to kilometers per hour	3.6
meters per second to meters per minute	0.0166667
meters per second to miles per hour	2.2336936
kilometers per hour to meters per second	0.2777778
kilometers per hour to meters per minute	16.666667
kilometers per hour to miles per hour	0.6213712
meters per minute to meters per second	60
meters per minute to kilometers per hour	0.06
meters per minute to miles per hour	0.0372823
miles per hour to meters per second	0.4470400
miles per hour to kilometers per hour	1.6093440
miles per hour to meters per minute	26.822400

it moved. A subject performs work while pedaling a cycle ergometer, which can be calculated by the force required to overcome the resistance against the flywheel times the distance that the flywheel traveled. A weightlifter who raises a barbell performs positive work, and negative work when he/she lowers the weight. However, by definition, no work is accomplished by the same weightlifter who holds the barbell steady above his/her head since there is no movement of the barbell. Neither is work performed by an individual running on a level treadmill as the subject is applying a vertical force while moving only horizontally. If the treadmill grade were raised, then the work performed would equal force times only the vertical distance traveled on the raised treadmill (Table 6).

Power is the rate of doing work. For example, a 100-kg individual who ran up the stadium stairs in the same time as a 50-kg individual generated twice as much power. The force applied by the heavier individual had to have been twice as great as that of the lighter individual in order to run the stairs in the same time (Table 7).

TABLE 5
Metric units of force and conversion factors.

SI unit	Equivalent metric unit	Equivalent English unit
Newton (N)	1 kilogram-meter per second per second (kg · m · s^{-2}) 0.101972 kiloponds (kp)	0.224809 pounds (lb)

To convert:	Multiply by:
Newtons to kiloponds	0.101972
kiloponds to Newtons	9.806650

TABLE 6
Metric units of work and conversion factors.

SI unit	Equivalent metric unit	Equivalent English unit
Joule (J)	1 Newton-meter (N · m) 1 kilopond-meter (kp · m) 0.2388459 calorie (cal)	9.4878134×10^{-4} British Thermal Units (BTU)

To convert:	Multiply by:
Joules to calories	0.2388459
calories to Joules	4.186780

ENERGY

Energy is another expression of work and exists in several forms. The chemical energy found in foods is converted by skeletal muscle into mechanical energy, which allows the joints to move. However, skeletal muscles are only approximately 25% efficient, so that about 75% of the chemical energy in foods is lost as another form of energy—heat—rather than being converted into mechanical energy. In exercise physiology, oxygen consumption ($\dot{V}O_2$) is frequently used as an indirect measure of energy (Table 8).

ABSOLUTE AND RELATIVE EXPRESSIONS

Units of measure can be expressed as an absolute expression or relative to an individual. Relative expressions, though, are frequently used in exercise physiology to allow easier comparisons between individuals. To illustrate this, consider the strength comparison between a 50-kg female and a 100-kg male. The maximal arm curl of the female is 25 kg and is 40 lb for the male. How would you answer the question of who is strongest? On the one hand, the

TABLE 7
Metric units of power and conversion factors.

SI unit	Equivalent metric unit	Equivalent English unit
Watt (W)	1 Joule per second (J · s⁻¹) 6.118 kilogram-meter per minute (kg · m· min⁻¹) 0.2388459 kilocalorie per second (kcal · s⁻¹)	0.00134102 horsepower (hp)

To convert:	Multiply by:
Watts to kilogram-meters per minute	6.118
Watts to kilocalories per second	0.2388459
kilogram-meters per minute to Watts	0.1635
kilocalories per second to Watts	4.1867800

TABLE 8
Metric units of energy and conversion factors.

SI unit	Equivalent metric unit	Equivalent English unit
Joule (J)	0.2388459 calorie (cal) ~0.0478 L of oxygen	9.478134×10^{-4} British Thermal Units (BTU)

To convert	Multiply by:
Joules to calories	0.2388459
calories to Joules	4.1868000
liters of oxygen to kilocalories	5

male is stronger as he can curl more weight than the female. From another perspective, though, the female is stronger because she can curl 50% of her body weight while the male can curl only 40% of his weight. In this example, the male has greater absolute strength, but the female has greater strength relative to body weight.

As another example, an aerobics class is composed of college age students and one 75-year-old student. To recommend that all the students exercise at a heart rate intensity of 160 bpm would be inappropriate and dangerous to the older student. The 160-bpm exercise recommendation is an absolute recommendation; rather, the instructor should recommend that students exercise at a heart rate intensity that is relative to their age-adjusted predicted maximal heart rate.

RATES OF METABOLIC AND CARDIOVASCULAR EXPRESSIONS

Several abbreviations for the rates of metabolic and cardiovascular variables are expressed as amounts per minute. In many of these cases, a raised dot is placed over the abbreviation. One common example is cardiac output, measured in units of liters per minute, properly abbreviated as $\dot{Q}$. Another common example is the rate of oxygen utilization, typically reported in units of milliliters of oxygen per kilogram body weight per minute, which is abbreviated as $\dot{V}O_2$.

WORKING WITH LABORATORY DATA

LEVELS OF SIGNIFICANCE AND ROUNDING

Sometimes, numbers need to be rounded. The general rule is that if the preceding number is 4 or less, the number should be rounded down; if it is 5 or greater, the number should be rounded up. In addition, the number of decimal places in which a number is expressed indicates the level of precision of the measurement. As an example, consider the problem of measuring the distance between two points and reporting it in units of kilometers. The distance was measured with an automobile odometer in units of miles, which had a precision of 0.1 mile. In this example, the distance was measured at 9.4 miles. The conversion factor of miles to kilometers is 1.609344 km · mile^{-1}, but the question remains as to how far the decimal place should be carried. A hand calculator computes the product as 15.1278336 km. However, this suggests that the level of precision was to the closest 0.0000001 km, or 0.000000062 miles. Certainly, an automobile odometer does not possess that level of precision; consequently, the distance in this example should be reported as 15 km, or at the most, 15.1 km.

a. Round 23.74551 to two significant digits. _____

b. Round 2483.475834 to one significant digit. _____

c. What is the significance of a number rounded to a certain decimal place?

UNIT CONVERSION

175 lb _____ kg   88.6 kg _____ lb

78 °F _____ °C   39.2 °C _____ °F

187.6 m · min^{-1} _____ mph   72.5 in _____ cm

PRACTICE CALCULATIONS (INCLUDE UNITS)

a. Calculate SV if $\dot{Q}$ = 10 L · min^{-1} and HR = 155 bpm? _____

Cardiac output ($\dot{Q}$) = Heart rate (HR) × Stroke volume (SV)

b. Calculate the breathing rate if TV = 2 L · breathe^{-1} and $\dot{V}E$ = 60 L · min^{-1}

_____

Tidal volume (TV) = Minute ventilation ($\dot{V}E$) ÷ Breathing rate

c. Predict $\dot{V}O_2$ if running speed = 8.5 mile · hr^{-1}? _____

$\dot{V}O_2$ (mL · kg^{-1} · min^{-1}) = Running speed (m · min^{-1}) ×
0.2 (mL · kg^{-1} · min^{-1} / m · min^{-1}) + 3.5 (mL · kg^{-1} · min^{-1})

d. Determine the percent body fat of a 19-year-old male whose sum of four skinfolds was 79 mm. _____

*Density = 1.1125025 − (0.0013125 × Sum) + (0.0000055 × Sum²)
− 0.0002440 × Age
% Body Fat = (495 ÷ Density) − 450*

RELATIVE VERSUS ABSOLUTE COMPARISONS

a. Describe the difference between an absolute and relative comparison. Why might one value be used over another?

b. The $\dot{V}O_{2max}$ of a 53.6-kg female and a 103.2-kg male were measured as 4.45 L · min^{-1} and 3.98 L · min^{-1}, respectively. What were their $\dot{V}O_{2max}$ values if expressed as mL · kg^{-1} · min^{-1}? Who had the higher absolute $\dot{V}O_{2max}$? the higher relative $\dot{V}O_{2max}$?

c. If the female subject ran a race at 60% of her $\dot{V}O_{2max}$, what was her $\dot{V}O_2$?

d. If the male subject ran a treadmill test at a $\dot{V}O_2$ of 25.44 mL · kg^{-1} · min^{-1}, what was his relative workload?

e. If an exercise prescription calls for 30 min of continuous exercise at 90% the maximal HR, what are the target heart rates for two 20-year-old individuals who have maximal HRs of 189 bpm and 206 bpm? Identify the absolute and relative HR intensities.

f. Explain the meaning of this statement: Females are equally as strong as males in lower body strength when strength is expressed per kilogram of fat-free body mass.

COMPONENTS OF A GRAPH

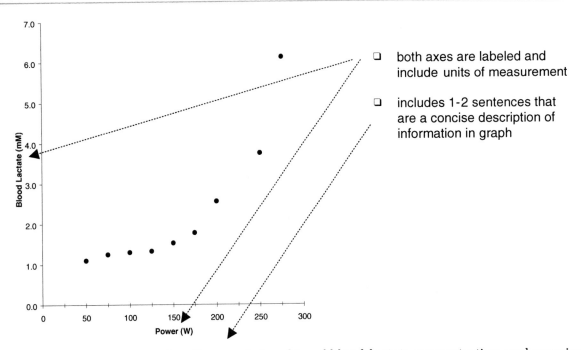

- both axes are labeled and include units of measurement

- includes 1-2 sentences that are a concise description of information in graph

FIGURE 1. Curvilinear relationship of blood lactate concentration and exercise intensity. The lactate threshold occurred at 175 W.

GRAPH CONSTRUCTION

A variable can be an *independent variable*, one that the investigator controls, or a *dependent variable*, the variable measured after manipulation of the independent variable. By convention, the independent variable is plotted on the X-axis (the horizontal coordinate or abscissa) with the dependent variable plotted on the Y-axis (the vertical component or ordinate).

After plotting, the relationship of the data needs to be interpreted. The most common relationships that are observed in exercise physiology are *linear* or *curvilinear* (alinear). In a linear relationship, the data would center on a line

TABLE 9
Data for Graph 1.

Heart Rate (bpm)	Workload (W)
98	50
112	70
142	125
167	175
179	190

TABLE 10
Data for Graph 2.

Blood Lactate (mmol · L^{-1})	Relative Workload (% of $\dot{V}O_{2max}$)
1.1	40
1.4	50
1.9	60
3.1	70
4.8	80
6.7	90

of best fit. Thus, if HR increased by a certain proportion with a 1 mph increase in treadmill speed, every subsequent 1 mph increase in speed would raise HR the same proportion. On the graph, the data would appear to be in a straight line. In a typical curvilinear relationship, there is little increase in the dependent variable at low exercise intensities until a certain point is reached when further increases in the intensity result in large increases in the dependent variable. The above graph illustrates a curvilinear relationship between blood lactate concentration and power output.

To see examples of these two relationships, construct two graphs using the data below (Tables 9 and 10). Be sure to properly label all parts of the graph. Also, rather than drawing lines that connect the data points, draw instead a line, or curve, of best fit through the data points and describe the type of relationship of each graph. Identify the dependent and independent variables in each graph.

Explain the information presented in the following graphs (Figures 2–4).

STATISTICAL SIGNIFICANCE

If one were to flip two pennies ten times each, and heads appeared seven times on one coin but only three times on the other coin, we would not readily conclude that the coins were different but that the difference occurred by chance. This illustrates the randomness associated with the taking of measurements, particularly with physiological measurements. If we measured body composition or $\dot{V}O_{2max}$ on a subject one day, most assuredly his/her per-

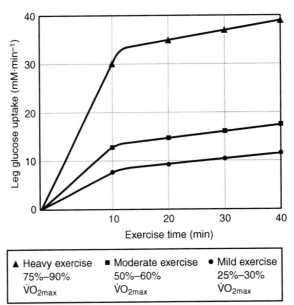

FIGURE 2. Adapted with permission from McArdle, W.D., F.I. Katch, and V.L. Katch. *Exercise Physiology: Energy, Nutrition, and Human Performance.* Philadephia: Lippincott Williams & Wilkins, 2001, Figure 1.5.

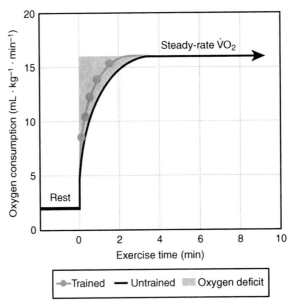

FIGURE 3. Adapted with permission from McArdle, W.D., F.I. Katch, and V.L. Katch. *Exercise Physiology: Energy, Nutrition, and Human Performance.* Philadephia: Lippincott Williams & Wilkins, 2001, Figure 7.3.

cent fat and $\dot{V}O_{2max}$ would be slightly different if we measured the subject later that day or the day after. Subject variations and measurement errors cause the inconsistencies observed with repeated measurements. In a specific example from a study on creatine supplementation, subjects assigned to the placebo group ran a 700 m time trial and averaged 108.1 s while subjects in the creatine group averaged 107.8 s for the distance[36]. However, statistical

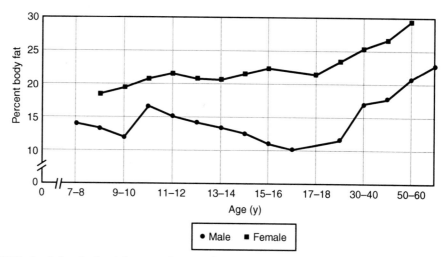

FIGURE 4. Adapted with permission from McArdle, W.D., F.I. Katch, and V.L. Katch. *Exercise Physiology: Energy, Nutrition, and Human Performance.* Philadephia: Lippincott Williams & Wilkins, 2001, Figure 31.13.

analysis suggested that the faster time by the creatine group was due not from the effect of creatine, but rather resulted from normal variations in performance. Thus, one should be careful to not interpret a difference between two means as actually having been caused by the treatment effect; rather, the difference may have been due merely to chance and normal subject variations. To compare the means of two or more trials, researchers perform a statistical analysis in order to determine whether there was a real difference or that it occurred simply by chance. In scientific papers and presentations, researchers indicate a statistical difference between two means by denoting one of the mean values with a symbol such as an asterisk. When viewing experimental results, one should always consider whether a statistical analysis was performed before determining whether any differences between means were truly different.

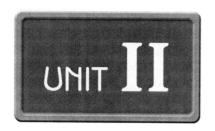

Cardiovascular Responses to Exercise

During exercise, primary roles of the cardiovascular system are to increase delivery of O_2 and nutrients to the working muscle as well as to carry away end-products of metabolism such as CO_2 and lactic acid. Two other important roles of the cardiovascular system are to dissipate excess heat produced during exercise and to deliver the catecholamines that regulate both the cardiovascular system and energy metabolism.

These functions are accomplished by movement of blood throughout the body, and although the body has more than enough blood for its needs at rest, it does not have sufficient blood during hard exercise. At rest, approximately two-thirds of the blood resides in the venous system as these vessels are much more compliant—the ability to stretch and hold blood—than the arterial blood vessels. With the onset of exercise, the circulatory system must prioritize the distribution of blood and redirect blood flow to the working muscles. This is accomplished by neural, hormonal, and local factors that change the vessel diameter to allow either an increase or decrease of blood flow through a tissue.

Blood flows through the circulatory system because of the pumping action by the heart. This is described by the cardiac output ($\dot{Q}$), which is the amount of blood pumped out in a minute ($L \cdot min^{-1}$), and can be calculated as the product of heart rate (HR) and stroke volume (SV). Three variables influence SV: *preload*, *afterload*, and *myocardial contractility*. Preload is the volume of blood in the left ventricle at the end of diastole—when the heart has finished filling and is about to contract. Venous return and plasma volume affect preload; for example, a larger preload results in a greater SV. Afterload is the resistance (i.e., aortic blood pressure) that the heart must overcome in order to eject the blood from the ventricle. Blood present in the aorta exerts a pressure and in order for the left ventricle to eject the blood, it must pressurize the blood in the left ventricle in excess of the aortic blood pressure (BP). Thus, when aortic BP is abnormally high, as during hypertension, the heart is forced to contract even harder to overcome the elevated aortic BP before blood can be ejected.

Although the heart is regulated through intrinsic means, the primary mechanisms during exercise are from the dual innervation of the sympathetic and parasympathetic divisions of the autonomic nervous system. The pair of vagus nerves, which originate in a cardioinhibitory center of the medulla oblongata, carry parasympathetic nerves that innervate the SA and AV nodes of the heart. When stimulated, parasympathetic nerve endings release acetylcholine that decreases the rate at which the nodes generate action potentials, thus decreasing HR. Sympathetic nerve endings release norepinephrine and have an opposite effect to that of parasympathetic innervation. Not only are the SA and AV nodes innervated by sympathetic nerves, but the myocardium is innervated as well, which increases both HR and myocardial contractility. During exercise, sympathetic stimulation predominates over parasympathetic inhibition, hence the heart is under primarily sympathetic control.

The arterial and venous blood vessels are also under sympathetic innervation. Sympathetic stimulation of the vascular smooth muscle results in vasoconstriction, which increases the resistance to blood flow thereby reducing flow. As compliance of the venous blood vessels is much greater than the arterial vessels, constriction of the venous vessels reduces the blood that can be in the vessel and results in an increased venous return. Assisting in venous return are the numerous one-way valves located within the veins that prevent blood from flowing back into the tissues. In addition, venous return is aided by rhythmic muscular contractions, such as during running or cycling, in which the blood is forced back to the heart.

The lab activities in this section investigate the response of the cardiovascular system to exercise. In addition, the virtual lab activities investigate the regulation and control of the cardiovascular system during exercise.

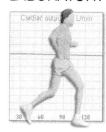

Heart Rate and Blood Pressure Response to Exercise

STUDENT ACTIVITY INVESTIGATION   Name_____

PURPOSE

With the onset of exercise, oxygen needs increase dramatically by the working muscle. In order to increase oxygen availability to working muscles, a number of changes must occur within the cardiovascular system. The purpose of this lab is to investigate the effects of exercise intensity on the HR and BP responses.

METHODS

1. Form groups of three or four students. Practice taking HR and BP on each other until everyone is able to perform these measurements accurately. See *Standardized Steps in Blood Pressure Measurement* (Appendix J) for guidelines on measuring BP. For HR measurement, palpate the radial or carotid pulse with the first and second fingers; count the pulses for at least a 30-s period and then convert the count to beats per minute. Shorter measurement times increase the likelihood of error in the HR. Also, check with your instructor to be sure that resistance of the cycle ergometer has been properly calibrated. If telemetry HR monitors are available (e.g., Polar HR monitors), use these also to check accuracy of the palpation measurements.

2. At least two subjects in each group should perform the exercise. Test additional subjects as time permits. Adjust the seat height of the cycle ergometer to get a proper knee angle; the seat height should allow the leg to be at near full extension (5-10°) when the foot is at the bottom of the pedal.

3. The subject will perform what is termed a *discontinuous graded exercise test* in which the subject performs repeated cycling bouts that increase in intensity and are separated by brief rest periods. First, take resting HR and BP measurements. Then, have the subject pedal for 4 min at 60 rpm with the cycle loaded to 1 kg of resistance (60 W of power). Constantly monitor the pedaling frequency to ensure that the subject is pedaling at the prescribed frequency. Otherwise, power output will be altered which will affect the data. During the last minute of the bout, measure and record HR and BP. If you have problems measuring HR or BP, have the subject continue pedaling until obtaining the data. In between bouts, allow the subject to rest for

1-3 min. For each subsequent bout, increase the resistance by 30 W (raising the resistance by 0.5-kg increments) until reaching 240 W or until the subject can no longer maintain a pedaling frequency of 60 rpm due to fatigue.

4. Mean the HR and BP data for each measurement. Graph both HR and BP on the same graph. Place the HR scale on the left Y-axis and the BP scale on the right Y-axis. Use different colors or symbols to differentiate the three data points. Be sure that the graph is appropriately labeled.

QUESTIONS

1. *Explain why measurements of HR and BP were taken during the last minute of an exercise bout rather than at the beginning of a bout.*

2. *Describe the relationship, and its shape, of exercise intensity and the HR response.*

3. *Predict the effect of increasing exercise intensity on $\dot{Q}$. What data do you have that would lend support to your hypothesis? Explain.*

4. *Contrast the effect of exercise intensity on the systolic and diastolic BP responses.*

LABORATORY **2**

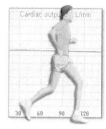

Cardiovascular Responses to Exercise

STUDENT ACTIVITY INVESTIGATION

Name_____

RESEARCH QUESTION

The research questions are to investigate the effects of exercise intensity on HR and BP responses as well as to compare the responses from dynamic (e.g., cycling) to that from maximal isometric exercise (e.g., handgrip dynamometer). Form groups of 3-4 students, and as a group, develop an experimental design to answer the research questions. After completing the data collection, prepare appropriate graphs that illustrate your results and respond to the italicized questions.

CONSIDERATIONS FOR DESIGNING THE EXPERIMENT

See *Standardized Steps in Blood Pressure Measurement* (Appendix J) for guidelines on measuring BP. Be sure to practice these skills prior to beginning data collection. During a test, if you have trouble with taking BP, repeat the measurement until you obtain reasonable values! If measuring HR with palpation of the pulse, count the pulses for at least a 30-s period and then convert the count to beats per minute. Shorter measurement times increase the likelihood of error in the HR measurement. Another consideration is to be sure that HR and BP have achieved a steady state before taking a measurement as any measurements taken before reaching steady state would not be valid. Although the treadmill is a common ergometer for exercise testing, they often are so noisy as to make listening for BP sounds difficult. A better alternative would be to use a cycle ergometer and to have the subject remove his/her arm from the handlebars when taking BP.

QUESTIONS

1. *Explain why measurements of HR and BP were not taken until the last minute of an exercise bout rather than earlier in the bout.*

CARDIOVASCULAR RESPONSES TO EXERCISE   17

2. *Describe the relationship, and its shape, of exercise intensity and the HR response.*

3. *Predict the effect of increasing exercise intensity on $\dot{Q}$. What data do you have that would lend support to your hypothesis? Explain.*

4. *Contrast the effect of exercise intensity on the systolic and diastolic BP responses.*

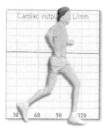

LABORATORY **3**

Cardiovascular Responses to Prolonged Exercise in the Heat

STUDENT ACTIVITY INVESTIGATION   Name_____

Humans are only about 25% efficient converting the chemical energy in food to mechanical energy for movement; the remaining energy is lost as heat. In order to ensure that the body temperature remains within a narrow range of 37 to 40 °C (98 to 104 °F), the body regulates body temperature and dissipates extra heat into the environment. Essentially, body temperature is the equilibrium of factors that add and subtract body heat. Four mechanisms used to dissipate heat into the environment are:

- *Conduction* — transfer of heat through direct contact,

- *Convection* — transfer of heat through air or liquid as is passes over the body,

- *Radiation* — transfer of heat through electromagnetic rays, and

- *Evaporation* — transfer of heat to convert liquid water to a vapor.

While resting in moderate ambient conditions, the metabolic rate is low enough so that the magnitude of excess heat is low. The body easily dissipates most of the extra heat through radiation. However, during exercise, the metabolic rate is increased many times and is more than can be dissipated by only radiation. Consequently, during exercise the body relies primarily on evaporation to maintain thermobalance.

Maintaining thermobalance while exercising in extreme environmental conditions is difficult. As air temperature increases, the ability to dissipate excess heat via radiation decreases and will even stop if air temperature becomes greater than skin temperature. Humidity also affects thermoregulation. The presence of water vapor in air decreases the ability of sweat to evaporate. When the relative humidity (RH) is 100%, the air is saturated with water vapor and thus, sweat evaporation cannot occur. Consequently, heat dissipation during exercise on a day with a high air temperature and RH is difficult.

There are two water compartments in the body: the *intracellular fluid* (ICF) and the *extracellular fluid* (ECF) compartments. Approximately 60-65% of the water is in the ICF as it supports cell form and structure as well as providing a medium for metabolism. The ECF is comprised of the interstitial fluid, which surrounds the cells, and the blood plasma, lymph, and other fluids. Transport of nutrients and waste products occurs via the ECF.

As one sweats, a large portion of water loss is primarily from the ECF, which decreases blood volume and in turn SV. Consequently, HR will increase to maintain cardiac output in order to meet the demands of exercise. Additionally, excessive sweat loss triggers the release of antidiuretic hormone (ADH) causing the kidneys to reduce urine production and conserve body water.

The amount of water lost during exercise can be closely determined by taking pre- and post-exercise weights. Moreover, the amount of energy loss from sweat evaporation can be estimated from the total water loss (1 L of evaporated sweat = 580 kcal).

PURPOSE

The purpose of this lab is to investigate the physiological effects of exercising in a hot environment. This is a 2-week experiment in which subjects will perform the same 30-min cycling bout each week but under different conditions, one being in a simulated hot environment and the other performed in a normal room temperature.

METHODS

Form groups of 3-4 students. At least two students from each group will serve as a subject, but test more as time permits. One trial will be performed with the subject wearing only running shorts and a T-shirt; the other trial will be a simulated heat trial in which the subjects wears extra clothing (e.g., long sleeve shirts, sweatshirts, sweatpants, woolen caps, gloves). Note: Caution should be followed in testing subjects in the heat trial. If a subject begins showing signs of heat stress, such as extreme fatigue or weakness, cessation of sweating, chills, pale or clammy skin, the exercise should be terminated and the subject immediately cooled down. For the first week, one subject should exercise in the control (room temperature) condition and the other in the simulated hot condition.

1. Record baseline measures of body weight, BP, HR, and hematocrit (Hct). If possible, move the scale into a small, private room/office and have the subject take a nude weight of him-/herself. Either you or the instructor will perform Hct measurements. See *Measuring Blood Lactate Concentration and Hematocrit* (Appendix K) for guidelines on sampling blood for Hct measurements.

2. Adjust seat height of the cycle ergometer so that the knee angle is at a 10-15° when the pedal is at the bottom.

3. Estimate 60% of each subject's HR_{max}. Have the subject select a comfortable pedaling frequency (e.g., 60-80 rpm) and begin increasing the resistance until the subject's HR approximates 60% of his/her HR_{max}. HR will take 2-3 min to reach a steady state, so make small increases in the cycle resistance so not to overshoot the intended intensity. After 5-6 min, do not adjust workload anymore unless the subject begins to fatigue and would otherwise not be able to complete the bout. Record the time and magnitude of changes to the resistance that were made so that the second trial can be performed exactly as the first. Record the final power output as well. Throughout the test, monitor the subject's pedaling frequency to ensure that he/she is maintaining the prescribed power output.

4. Measure and record HR, BP, and rating of perceived exertion (RPE), every 10 min of the 30-min cycling bout.

5. Upon finishing the exercise bout, record the subject's post-exercise weight and measure the post-exercise Hct.

6. Average responses from all subjects from each of the two conditions and record the means in Table 3.1 below.

7. On separate graphs, plot the means of the two conditions against time for HR, BP, and RPE.

QUESTIONS

1. *Calculate the sweat rate for each trial and compare.* (Note: One liter of sweat weighs approximately 1 kg.)

   Sweat rate $(L \cdot hr^{-1})$ = [Weight$_{pre}$ (kg) - Weight$_{post}$ (kg)] ÷ Exercise duration (hr)

2. *Calculate the percentage change in plasma volume (PV) for each trial using the van Beaumont et al. equation[38].*

   $$\%\Delta PV = [100 \div (100\text{-Hct}_{pre})] \times [(100 \times (\text{Hct}_{pre} - \text{Hct}_{post})) \div \text{Hct}_{post}]$$

Table 3.1

	Control Trial		Hot Trial	
Date				
Lab temperature (°C)				
Relative humidity (%)				
Power (W)				

Time (min)	Lost weight (kg)		Hematocrit (%)		HR (bpm)		BP (mm Hg)		RPE	
	Control	Hot	Control	Hot	Control	Hot	Control	Hot	Control	Hot
0							/	/		
10							/	/		
20							/	/		
30							/	/		

3. *Offer an explanation for the changes in PV in relation to the calculated sweat rates for the two trials.* Support the hypothesis with your data.

4. Changes in blood flow to the skin affects the volume of blood pooled in the cutaneous vessels such that more blood is diverted to the cutaneous blood vessels. This decreases the amount of blood returning to the heart (i.e., venous return), thus reducing SV. *Assuming that $\dot{Q}$ remained the same during both trials, predict the effect that exercising in the hot condition should have on the exercise HR. Explain. Does your HR data support this hypothesis?*

5. In the heat, the body has a more difficult time in dissipating the excess heat produced during exercise. One mechanism that helps the body to dissipate heat is the vasodilation of cutaneous blood vessels. This allows heat produced in the body to be transported to the skin surface where part of the heat can be radiated to the environment. The increased vasodilation also decreases the total peripheral resistance (TPR) to blood flow. Blood pressure is the product of $\dot{Q}$ and TPR. Thus, a decrease in TPR would result in a lower BP response. *How should the BP responses between the two trials have compared? Did the data support your hypothesis?*

6. *What additional evidence can you provide that supports one trial being more stressful than the other trial?*

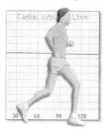

Cardiovascular Responses to Prolonged Exercise

VIRTUAL LAB INVESTIGATION

Name_____

PURPOSE

Soon after the onset of submaximal, but constant-intensity exercise, the physiological systems achieve steady state. Within 2-3 min, measures such as HR and $\dot{V}O_2$ become stable. However, as duration of the exercise becomes longer, the exercise becomes more stressful and a number of physiological changes occur gradually that influence many metabolic and cardiorespiratory parameters. The purpose of this laboratory activity is to investigate the effects of prolonged exercise on the cardiovascular system and potential mechanisms that explain these responses.

METHODS

There will be two exercise trials in this investigation. For the initial trial, select the female endurance athlete and have her perform a prolonged treadmill test at 21 °C and at sea level. Measure the following variables:

Cardiovascular measures

- cardiac output ($\dot{Q}$) including HR and SV
- blood pressures (SBP, DPB, MAP)
- skin and splanchnic blood flows
- total peripheral resistance (TPR)

Blood measures

- catecholamines (EPI and NE)

Thermoregulation

- Core temperature

Have the subject run for 3 h and take measurements at 10 min and every 30-min period thereafter. Afterwards, answer the italicized questions.

HEMODYNAMIC RESPONSES

1. Review the HR data. *Describe the effect of prolonged exercise on HR. Does this response seem strange even though treadmill speed remained constant?*

2. Review the $\dot{Q}$ data. *Describe the effect of prolonged exercise on $\dot{Q}$.*

3. Review the SV data. *What must be happening to SV to explain the HR and $\dot{Q}$ responses?*

4. Three variables that affect SV are: 1) preload (filling pressure), which is greatly influenced by venous return, 2) myocardial contractility (strength of contraction), and 3) afterload (the arterial BP that must be overcome by the heart in order to eject blood). *Because of the SV response, what must be occurring to venous return (the amount of blood returning to the heart)?*

BLOOD FLOW REDISTRIBUTION

5. Skin blood vessels are very compliant (meaning that they stretch easily and are able to accommodate a larger volume of blood). Therefore, changes in blood flow to the skin affects the volume of blood pooled in the cutaneous vessels. Review the skin blood flow responses. *What changes, if*

any, are occurring to the distribution of blood? How might this response affect venous return?

6. Since there is a limited supply of blood, and skin blood flow has changed, *predict the response of splanchnic blood flow. Explain the rationale for this change.* Confirm your prediction from the splanchnic blood flow data.

BLOOD PRESSURE REGULATION

7. Mean arterial blood pressure is a function of systolic and diastolic blood pressures (MAP = ⅓ SBP + ⅔DBP). MAP can also be calculated via Ohm's Law (MAP = $\dot{Q}$ × total peripheral resistance [TPR]). Review the blood pressure data. *Describe the effect of prolonged exercise on the blood pressure responses.*

8. Predict the response of TPR over time. Confirm your prediction from the TPR data. *Explain the response of TPR as it relates to blood flow redistribution during the exercise bout.*

PHYSIOLOGICAL MECHANISMS

9. In response to physical or psychological stress, the body responds with a general sympathetic stimulation. This results in the release of catecholamines, epinephrine (EPI) and norepinephrine (NE), from the adrenal medulla. The catecholamines impact a number of physiological systems, and their effects include increased HR, myocardial contractility, and peripheral vasoconstriction. Review the plasma catecholamine responses. Predict the effect of catecholamines on the splanchnic blood vessels and

flow. *How did the release of catecholamines affect splanchnic blood flow during the exercise bout?*

10. Catecholamines also cause vasoconstriction in the cutaneous vessels. However, because the body is only ~25% efficient, heat builds up during exercise. This is sensed by the hypothalamus, which in turn signals the cutaneous vessels to dilate in order to dissipate the additional heat. Consequently, skin blood flow increases, and as previously learned, blood pools in the periphery, thus decreasing venous return. This reduces preload to the heart leading to a decrease in SV. In order for $\dot{Q}$ to be maintained, HR must increase, thus the occurrence of cardiovascular drift.

Repeat the exercise trial with the same subject, but perform the exercise instead at 33 °C and with no fluids administered during exercise. Data from the second trial will overlay that from the first trial. Before you begin the second trial, however, predict how the following responses in the hot environment will compare to those at room temperature.

- HR and SV
- MAP
- core temperature
- skin and splanchnic blood flows
- plasma [EPI]

11. *Discuss the differences in the responses of these variables between the two trials. Include discussion on a potential mechanism that explains these differences.*

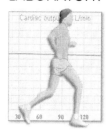

Training Effects on Cardiovascular Responses to Prolonged Exercise

VIRTUAL LAB INVESTIGATION

Name_____

PURPOSE

The purpose of this study is to investigate the cardiovascular adaptations that occur from endurance running. Initially, a sedentary female will perform a prolonged treadmill test during which a number of cardiovascular parameters will be measured. The exercise test will be repeated with the same individual, but after she has been training for about a year.

METHODS

First, select the sedentary female and take resting measurements of the variables listed below. Have her perform a prolonged treadmill test for 60 min at 115 m · min^{-1}, 21 °C, and at sea level. Measure these variables at 10 min and every 30 min period. Repeat the exercise trial at the same speed and conditions, but instead test the trained female (not the female endurance athlete). After her training, she will now be able to run for 90 min. Afterwards, answer the italicized questions.

The trained subject is the same individual as the sedentary but after having had endurance training for about a year. Because of her training, her maximal aerobic uptake ($\dot{V}O_{2max}$) increased from 37.2 to 44.5 mL · kg^{-1} · min^{-1}. Often times, exercise intensities are determined relative to one's $\dot{V}O_{2max}$. Note that in this part of the investigation, the two trials are being performed at the same absolute intensities. However, as is discussed later, during the trained trial the subject will be running at a lower relative intensity, relative to her $\dot{V}O_{2max}$.

Measure the following variables:

Cardiovascular measures

- cardiac output ($\dot{Q}$) including HR and SV
- skin and splanchnic blood flows

Blood measures

- plasma volume
- catecholamines (EPI and NE)

Pulmonary measures

- $\dot{V}O_2$

Additional measures

- Rating of perceived exertion (RPE)

RESTING RESPONSES

1. In response to stress/overload, cardiac muscle hypertrophy is similar to skeletal muscle hypertrophy. With endurance training, cardiac muscle hypertrophy results in an increased left ventricular chamber, which allows for greater stroke volumes. Review the resting HR, SV, and $\dot{Q}$ data from both trials. *What effect did training have on the body's need for cardiac output while at rest?* The cardiac output is the product of HR and SV. *How were the two determinants of cardiac output affected by training? Suggest a mechanism to explain this adaptation.*

2. *Predict how this adaptation will affect HR and SV during exercise.*

EXERCISE INTENSITY

3. Both trials were performed at the same absolute exercise intensity, 115 m · min^{-1}. However, exercise intensity is often expressed relative to $\dot{V}O_{2max}$. Divide the 30-min $\dot{V}O_2$ values by the subject's respective $\dot{V}O_{2max}$ and express this ratio as a percentage. *How hard was the subject running during each trial relative to her $\dot{V}O_{2max}$ at the time of the measurement?*

4. Review the RPE for the two trials. *What effect might the difference in relative exercise intensity between the two trials have had on the endurance performance? How does the RPE data support your response?*

HEMODYNAMIC ADAPTATIONS

5. Review the exercise HR, SV, and $\dot{Q}$ data for the two trials. *What effect did training have on the body's need for cardiac output during exercise? How did training affect HR and SV during exercise?*

6. *Describe the effect of training on the resting and exercise HR and SV. How can the effect of exercise training on cardiac hypertrophy help to explain these adaptations?*

7. The release of catecholamines (epinephrine and norepinephrine) has numerous effects in the body, including stimulation of the cardiovascular system. One of the most well known effects is stimulation of the sinoatrial (SA) node in the heart, which results in higher heart rates. Review the exercise catecholamine data. *Describe the relationship of catecholamines to the HR responses between the two trials.*

8. Another well-known effect of the catecholamines on the cardiovascular system is that they promote vasoconstriction in most vascular beds. *Predict the effect of training on splanchnic blood flow. Explain the reasoning for your prediction.* To corroborate your prediction, review the splanchnic blood flows from the two trials.

9. Preload to the heart is also influenced by plasma volume. Compare resting PV between the two trials. *How might this difference help to explain the differences in SV between the two trials?*

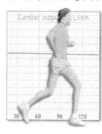

Cardiovascular Responses to Graded Exercise

VIRTUAL LAB INVESTIGATION   Name_____

PURPOSE

Soon after the onset of submaximal exercise, the physiological systems achieve steady state. Within 2-3 min, measures such as HR and $\dot{V}O_2$ become stable. However, as intensity of the exercise increases, the exercise becomes more stressful, which influences many metabolic and cardiorespiratory parameters. The purpose of this laboratory activity is to investigate the effects of graded exercise on the cardiovascular system and the potential mechanisms that explain these responses.

METHODS

Select the trained male and have him perform a graded treadmill test to exhaustion at 21°C and at sea level. Measure the following variables:

Cardiovascular measures

- cardiac output ($\dot{Q}$) including HR and SV
- blood pressures (SBP, DPB, MAP)
- total peripheral resistance (TPR)
- a-v O_2 diff
- muscle, skin, and splanchnic blood flows

Blood measures

- catecholamines (EPI and NE)

Pulmonary measures

- Oxygen uptake ($\dot{V}O_2$)

Have the subject run to exhaustion during a graded exercise bout in which treadmill speed is increased 25 m · min^{-1} (~0.9 miles · hr^{-1}) every 3 min. Afterwards, answer the italicized questions.

HEMODYNAMIC RESPONSES

1. Review the HR data. *Describe the relationship, including its shape, of exercise intensity on HR.*

2. Review the SV data. *Describe the relationship, including its shape, of exercise intensity on SV.*

3. Review the $\dot{Q}$ response and compare it to the HR and SV data. *Describe the relationship, including its shape, of exercise intensity on $\dot{Q}$.*

4. The three variables that affect SV are: 1) preload (filling pressure), which is greatly influenced by venous return, 2) myocardial contractility (strength of contraction), and 3) afterload (the arterial BP that must be overcome by the heart in order to eject blood). *Because of the SV response, what must be occurring to venous return (the amount of blood returning to the heart) as exercise intensity increases?*

BLOOD FLOW REDISTRIBUTION

5. As treadmill speed increases, more work is required of the leg muscles. Thus, the oxygen demands of working muscles are increased so that more ATP can be resynthesized. *Predict the effect of exercise intensity on muscle blood flow.* Plot muscle blood flow against treadmill speed. Since there is a

limited supply of blood, and muscle blood flow has changed, *predict the response of splanchnic blood flow. Explain the reasoning for this change.* Review the splanchnic blood flow and compare it to the muscle blood flow data.

BLOOD PRESSURE REGULATION

6. Mean arterial blood (MAP) pressure is a function of systolic (SBP) and diastolic (DBP) blood pressures (MAP = $\frac{1}{3}$ SBP + $\frac{2}{3}$ DBP). According to Ohm's Law, MAP can also be calculated using the following: MAP = $\dot{Q}$ × total peripheral resistance (TPR). On a single graph, plot SBP, DBP, and MAP against treadmill speed. Print out the graph. *Describe the effect of exercise intensity on the systolic and diastolic blood pressure responses.*

PHYSIOLOGICAL MECHANISMS

7. Review the $\dot{Q}$ data. Approximately, how many fold increase of $\dot{Q}$ was there from rest to maximal intensity? In light of Ohm's Law and the changes in $\dot{Q}$ and MAP with exercise intensity, how must have TPR responded? Review the TPR response. *Explain the response of TPR with increasing exercise intensity as it relates to blood flow redistribution.*

8. In response to physical or psychological stress, the body responds with a general sympathetic stimulation. This results in the release of catecholamines, epinephrine (EPI) and norepinephrine (NE), from the adrenal medulla. The catecholamines impact a number of physiological systems, and their effects include increased HR, myocardial contractility (i.e., SV), and peripheral vasoconstriction. Review the plasma catecholamine responses. Predict the effect of catecholamines on the splanchnic blood vessels and flow. *How did the release of catecholamines affect splanchnic blood flow during the exercise bout?*

9. Given the result of catecholamines on the smooth muscle surrounding blood vessels, working muscle must have some mechanism(s) to override

the vasoconstriction effect if it is to increase blood flow and oxygen delivery. As muscle is recruited for work, it becomes metabolically active which results in the accumulation of metabolic end products. These metabolites, such as H^+, adenosine, CO_2, K^+, and nitric oxide (NO), are known to be potent vasodilators that override the effects of catecholamines and sympathetic stimulation that result in increased local muscle blood flow.

MAXIMAL AEROBIC POWER

10. A primary purpose of blood flow to the working muscle is delivery of oxygen so that muscle can use the oxygen to re-synthesize ATP. The rate of oxygen utilization ($\dot{V}O_2$) is usually measured as an absolute value of liters of oxygen per minute ($L \cdot min^{-1}$) or relative to body weight as milliliters of oxygen per kilogram body weight per minute ($mL \cdot kg^{-1} \cdot min^{-1}$). At rest, $\dot{V}O_2$ is ~3.5 $mL \cdot kg^{-1} \cdot min^{-1}$ (~0.25 $L \cdot min^{-1}$). Predict the effect of exercise intensity on $\dot{V}O_2$. Review the $\dot{V}O_2$ data. The maximal rate at which the muscles can consume oxygen is termed $\dot{V}O_{2max}$. *Identify the subject's $\dot{V}O_{2max}$* (in $mL \cdot kg^{-1} \cdot min^{-1}$). Use information from Appendix I to evaluate the training status of your subject.

11. According to Fick's Law, $\dot{V}O_2$ is the product of three parameters: HR, SV, and a-v O_2 diff. The a-v O_2 diff, also known as oxygen extraction, is defined as the difference in oxygen content (expressed in milliliter of O_2 per 100 mL of blood) between arterial blood and the mixed venous blood. For example, if the HR was 72 bpm, SV was 70 $mL \cdot beat^{-1}$, the arterial oxygen content was 20 $mL \cdot 100 mL^{-1}$, and the mixed venous blood had an oxygen content of 15 $mL \cdot 100 mL^{-1}$, then

$$\dot{V}O_2 = HR \times SV \times \text{a-v } O_2 \text{ diff}$$

$$= 72 \frac{beats}{min} \times 70 \frac{mL}{beat} \times \frac{(20 - 15)\ mL}{100\ ml}$$

$$= 252\ mL \cdot min^{-1}\ (0.25\ L \cdot min^{-1})$$

12. With reference to the above equation, if $\dot{V}O_2$ was to increase with a rise in exercise intensity, HR, SV, or a-v O_2 diff, or a combination of the three variables, must increase. Review the HR and SV graph. *Offer one explanation as to why they responded as they did with increased exercise intensity.*

13. As exercise intensity increases, several changes occur at the local level, which influence the binding strength of oxygen to hemoglobin. With exercise, there is a decrease in the PO_2 in the working muscle along with a increase of the PCO_2. In addition, at higher exercise intensities, the muscle pH decreases and the temperature increases. All of these changes decrease the binding of oxygen. Plot the a-v O_2 diff against treadmill speed. *What do these data suggest regarding the amount of oxygen being released by the hemoglobin to muscle?*

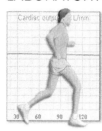

Training Effects on Cardiorespiratory Responses to Graded Exercise

VIRTUAL LAB INVESTIGATION

Name_____

PURPOSE

A number of cardiovascular and metabolic adaptations occur with endurance training. The purpose of this study is to investigate the cardiovascular adaptations that occur from endurance running. Initially, a male endurance athlete will perform a graded treadmill test during which a number of cardiovascular parameters will be measured. The exercise test will be repeated with the same individual after he has stopped running for about 6 months.

METHODS

Select the trained male and have him perform a graded treadmill test to exhaustion at 21°C and at sea level. Measure the following variables:

Cardiovascular measures

- cardiac output ($\dot{Q}$) including HR and SV
- blood pressures (SBP, DPB, MAP)
- total peripheral resistance (TPR)
- a-v O_2 diff
- muscle, skin, and splanchnic blood flows

Blood measures

- catecholamines (EPI and NE)

Pulmonary measures

- Oxygen uptake ($\dot{V}O_2$)

Have the subject run to exhaustion during a graded exercise bout in which treadmill speed is increased 25 m · min-1 every 3 min. Repeat the test under the same conditions, but using the detrained male endurance athlete. Afterwards, perform the requested data plots and answer the italicized questions.

HEMODYNAMIC RESPONSES

1. Review the $\dot{V}O_2$ data (in mL · kg^{-1} · min^{-1}) for both trials. Compare the $\dot{V}O_2$ values at the submaximal running speeds. *What does this comparison suggest about the effects of training on energy expenditure at submaximal exercise intensities?*

2. Compare the resting $\dot{V}O_2$ between the two trials as well as $\dot{Q}$. *What effect do these data suggest that endurance training had on the amount of oxygen needed by the body at rest?*

3. A training adaptation to the heart is that the chamber volumes, particularly the left ventricular volume, increase. *Predict the effect this has on SV.* Confirm your prediction by comparing the resting SVs.

4. *Based on the resting $\dot{Q}$ and the myocardial adaptations to training, predict the training effect on the resting HR.* Confirm your hypothesis by comparing the resting HRs.

5. Review the submaximal $\dot{Q}$ data from the two trials. *What effect do these data suggest that endurance training had on the amount of oxygen needed by the body during submaximal exercise?*

6. *Based on the resting SV data and the changes to left ventricular volume, predict the effect on SV at the submaximal intensities.* Confirm your hypothesis by comparing the submaximal exercise SV data between the two trials.

7. *Based on the submaximal exercise $\dot{Q}$ and SV responses, predict the effect of training on the HR response to submaximal exercise.* Confirm your hypothesis by comparing the submaximal exercise HR responses.

8. Compare the muscle capillary density between the two conditions. *Offer a rationale for why this adaptation might be of benefit. Predict the effect that this adaptation could have on the a-v O_2 diff.* Confirm your hypothesis by reviewing the a-v O_2 diff data of the two trials.

9. Compare the $\dot{V}O_{2max}$ values from the sedentary and trained trials. *What was the percent change in $\dot{V}O_{2max}$ following the endurance-training program?*

10. According to Fick's Law, $\dot{V}O_2$ is the product of three parameters: HR, SV, and a-v O_2 diff. The a-v O_2 diff, also known as oxygen extraction, is defined as the difference in oxygen content (expressed in milliliter of O_2 per 100 mL of blood) between arterial blood and the mixed venous blood. For example, if the HR was 72 bpm, SV was 70 mL $\cdot$ beat^{-1}, the arterial oxygen content was 20 mL $\cdot$ 100 mL^{-1}, and the mixed venous blood had a oxygen content of 15 mL $\cdot$ 100 mL^{-1}, then

$$\dot{V}O_2 = HR \times SV \times \text{a-v } O_2 \text{ diff}$$

$$= 72\,\frac{beats}{min} \times 70\,\frac{mL}{beat} \times \frac{(20-15)\,mL}{100\,mL}$$

$$= 252 \text{ mL} \cdot \text{min}^{-1}\ (0.25 \text{ L} \cdot \text{min}^{-1})$$

11. *Fill in Table 7-1 with the maximal data.*
Using data from above, what are the relative contributions of central hemodynamic ($\dot{Q}_{max}$) and peripheral changes (maximal a-v O_2 diff) in contributing to the training-induced adaptations in $\dot{V}O_{2max}$?

TABLE 7.1

	$\dot{V}O_{2max}$ (mL · kg^{-1} · min^{-1})	SV_{max} (mL · beat^{-1})	HR_{max} (beats · min^{-1})	$\dot{Q}_{max}$ (L · min^{-1})	maximal a-vO$_2$ diff (mL · 100 mL^{-1})
Detrained					
Trained					
% change					

12. As discussed in an earlier lab, catecholamines are released in response to exercise stress. Review the catecholamine responses of the two trials against treadmill speed (i.e., absolute workload). A method used in exercise physiology to equate submaximal workloads is to express the intensities relative to the maximal aerobic capacity ($\dot{V}O_{2max}$), i.e., $\dot{V}O_2$ expressed as a percentage of $\dot{V}O_{2max}$. Instead of using treadmill speed, plot the catecholamine responses against the workload expressed as a percentage of $\dot{V}O_{2max}$. For example if the $\dot{V}O_2$ at 135 m · min^{-1} were 30 mL · kg^{-1} · min^{-1} and the individual's $\dot{V}O_{2max}$ was 50 mL · kg^{-1} · min^{-1}, then the relative exercise intensity was 60% of the subject's $\dot{V}O_{2max}$. Further, if after training his $\dot{V}O_{2max}$ increased to 60 mL · kg^{-1} · min^{-1}, then the relative $\dot{V}O_2$ at 135 m · min^{-1} decreased to 50% of $\dot{V}O_{2max}$ while his absolute workload remained the same. (Note: training would have little or no effect on the energy expenditure ($\dot{V}O_2$) at submaximal running speeds.)

13. *Describe the differences of the absolute and relative sympathetic response to exercise.*

14. Sympathetic stimulation is known to decrease splanchnic blood flow. Predict the effect of training on splanchnic blood flow during submaximal exercise. Confirm your hypothesis from the splanchnic blood flow of the two conditions. Likewise, predict the training effect when splanchnic blood flow is plotted against the relative workload (i.e., expressed as a percentage of $\dot{V}O_{2max}$). *Describe the differences of the absolute and relative splanchnic blood flow response to exercise.*

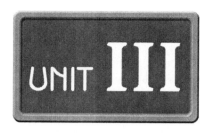

Metabolic Responses to Exercise

The carbohydrates and fats in the foods we ingest contain energy, and through metabolic reactions that take place in muscle, that energy is converted into mechanical energy for movement. Contraction of muscle requires energy in the form of adenosine triphosphate (ATP) not only by the myosin heads but also by the Na-K exchange pumps and Ca^{2+} pumps on the sarcoplasmic reticulum. The Na-K exchange pumps use ATP to maintain the Na^+ and K^+ concentration gradients across the cell membrane. In addition, myosin heads use ATP to detach from the actin filaments, and the Ca^{2+} pumps use ATP to remove Ca^{2+} from the sarcoplasm to the sarcoplasmic reticulum when excitation of the muscle fiber has ended. Moreover, the Ca^{2+} pumps have been estimated to use up to 30% of the total ATP synthesized during high-speed contractions.

Muscles store little ATP so that when excitation-contraction of the fibers begins, three metabolic energy pathways in muscle quickly replenish ATP. These energy pathways, ATP-phosphocreatine (PCr, which is also referred to as creatine phosphate), (anaerobic) glycolysis, and oxidative phosphorylation (aerobic), differ in the amount and rate at which they produce ATP.

Aerobic metabolism uses carbohydrates and fats as fuel, which occurs mostly in slow-twitch fibers. Carbohydrates from blood glucose and liver and muscle glycogen are partially oxidized through glycolysis into pyruvate, which then enters the Krebs' cycle (citric acid cycle) in the mitochondria as acetyl Coenzyme A. Fatty acids are also converted into acetyl Coenzyme A through a process called beta-oxidation. The Krebs' cycle occurs in the mitochondrial matrix where reducing equivalents (NAD and FAD) remove H^+ and electrons from the substrates. The reducing equivalents carry the H^+ and electrons to the electron transport chain located at the inner mitochondrial membrane. Here, the electrons are passed down a series of oxidative reactions catalyzed by the cytochrome enzymes in which the final electron acceptor is oxygen. During these reactions, H^+ is pumped out of the inner mitochondrial membrane, which creates electric and concentration gradients with the mitochondrial matrix. At some point, the H^+ diffuse back into the mitochondrial matrix, and the energy created by the return of H⁺ is captured to rephosphorylate ADP into ATP. Although some ATP is synthesized during glycolysis and the Krebs' cycle, the majority of ATP is synthesized in this step.

Even though the aerobic system can synthesize considerable ATP, it cannot synthesize ATP quickly enough to meet the muscle's demands during high-intensity activity. Moreover, mitochondria take 2-3 min to become fully activated after exercise begins. Thus, at the beginning of exercise and for high-intensity activities, muscles require other energy pathways to meet the ATP demand. During these times, glycolysis makes important contributions to ATP production. This energy pathway, the same as used by the aerobic system, synthesizes only 2-3 ATP from one glucose molecule, but the rate of glycolysis is so rapid that a considerable amount of ATP can be quickly synthesized during times of high-intensity exercise. However, instead of entering the mitochondria, most of the pyruvate is converted to lactate, and due in large part to the inhibitory effects of acidosis on glycolysis and glycogenolysis, the capacity for ATP production by glycolysis is small compared to aerobic metabolism.

However, glycolysis, in spite of its ability to rapidly synthesize ATP, requires several seconds to reach peak ATP production. With the onset of exercise, ATP demands increase immediately, thus another energy pathway is needed until glycolysis and the aerobic system are able to synthesize sufficient ATP. What is sometimes referred to as the "immediate" energy system, PCr transfers its high-energy phosphate to an ADP to synthesize ATP. The capacity of PCr to synthesize ATP is even smaller than glycolysis and limits its contribution to the initial 20-30 s of exercise, most of which is during the first few seconds.

A common misconception among some students of exercise physiology is that these energy pathways work in series such that PCr produces all the ATP for the first 20-30 s of exercise until it becomes exhausted, then glycolysis produces all the ATP for the next 2-3 min, which is followed by the aerobic system. Rather, at the onset of exercise, all three systems are synthesizing ATP although their contribution changes as the exercise progresses (Figure III-1).

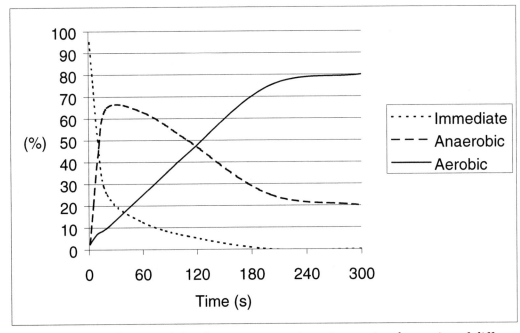

FIGURE III-1. Contribution of the three energy systems to maximal exercise of different durations.

Within the first few seconds of exercise, regardless of the intensity, PCr is contributing most of the ATP. From 5-8 s through 90-120 s, glycolysis contributes most of the ATP after which aerobic metabolism synthesizes the majority of ATP.

The series of experiments in this section investigate the interaction of these systems during exercise. In addition, the *Virtual Exercise Physiology Laboratory* activities investigate mechanisms that regulate the energy pathways and their utilization of fuels.

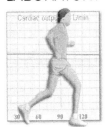

Measuring Energy Expenditure: Indirect Calorimetery

LAB DEMONSTRATION   Name_____

One characteristic of living animals is that they all give off heat. As a result of cellular respiration and cellular work, heat is produced. An operational definition of metabolism is the rate of heat production, which describes the metabolic rate.

$$\text{food} + O_2 \xrightarrow{\text{respiration}} \text{heat} + \text{ATP} \xrightarrow{\text{work}} \text{heat}$$

The direct measure of heat production, called direct calorimetry, is a technically difficult problem for human research so an alternative method is to measure the rate of oxygen consumed or utilized by the body for aerobic ATP production. The determination of the metabolic rate from the measure of oxygen consumption is called *indirect calorimetry.*

The development of gas analyzers in the 1960s and personal computers in the 1970s greatly enhanced the efficiency for making these measurements. In exercise physiology laboratories, metabolic measurement systems are utilized for indirect calorimetry measurement, which is termed open-circuit spirometry. Most systems measure the total volume of expired air, though a few systems instead measure inspiratory volume, as well as differences of oxygen and carbon dioxide levels from ambient and expired air. The system's computer uses this information to calculate the volumes of oxygen uptake ($\dot{V}O_2$) and carbon dioxide production ($\dot{V}CO_2$).

In order to take these measurements, a subject is fitted with a low-resistance, two-way non-rebreathing valve in her/his mouth, which directs all expired air to the metabolic measurement system via a long flexible hose (Figure 8.1).

As the expiratory air enters the system, it passes through a pneumotachometer, which measures air volume. Air from the pneumotachometer then enters a mixing chamber. At the beginning of expiration, composition of the air is higher in O_2 and lower in CO_2 than at the end of expiration. Thus, the air must be mixed together so that a representative sample can be taken. A sampling line connected to the mixing chamber draws a small volume of air to the oxygen and carbon dioxide analyzers that are interfaced, along with the pneumotachometer, to a computer.

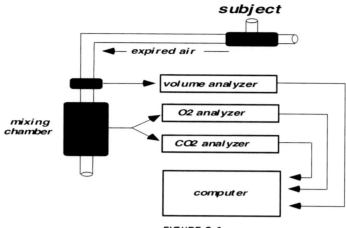

FIGURE 8-1.

As mentioned above, the amount of oxygen utilized is also a reflection of the energy expenditure and is sometimes expressed in units of kilojoules (kJ) or kilocalories (kcal). From previous research, approximately 5 kcal of energy are utilized for every liter of oxygen consumed. Thus, a subject who has consumed 2.5 L of oxygen during 10 min of quiet sitting would have expended 12.5 kcal, which is about the same amount of energy from a single French fry.

The metabolic rate is affected by numerous factors, and is always fluctuating. Activity or exercise will temporarily increase—up to 20X or more—the metabolic rate as will stress, illness, certain drugs and hormones, and the digestion and absorption of food. During exercise, however, these factors have little influence on the metabolic rate. Thus, to improve the accuracy of the resting metabolic rate (RMR), a subject must refrain from eating and exercising prior to the measurement.

PURPOSE

Using indirect calorimetry, the RMR (i.e., $\dot{V}O_2$) will be measured of a subject who has been sitting quietly. Afterwards, the subject will jog at a moderate pace (160 m · s^{-1} / 6 mph) for 5 min. The experiment will be repeated using a subject having a much different body weight. Afterwards, the $\dot{V}O_2$ values are to be compared (Table 8.1).

TABLE 8.1

	Subject 1		Subject 2	
	Weight (kg) _____		Weight (kg) _____	
	Sitting	Jogging	Sitting	Jogging
$\dot{V}O_2$ (mL · min^{-1})				
$\dot{V}O_2$ (mL · kg^{-1} · min^{-1})				

QUESTIONS

1. Provide several reasons for measuring $\dot{V}O_2$.

2. Explain why $\dot{V}O_2$ changed after going from sitting to jogging.

3. Compare $\dot{V}O_2$, expressed as $mL \cdot min^{-1}$, between the two subjects while they were sitting. While jogging. Provide a reason for the difference. Suggest an alternative expression of $\dot{V}O_2$ to better compare energy expenditure between individuals of differing body mass.

4. Predict how an increase of the exercise intensity would affect $\dot{V}O_2$.

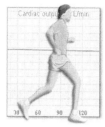

Oxygen Deficit and EPOC

LAB DEMONSTRATION

Name_____

One purpose for observing the metabolic response to exercise is to estimate the energy cost of the exercise for which indirect calorimetry is the method most frequently used. Recall that this method assumes all of the energy expended for the exercise is reflected by the magnitude of oxygen uptake ($\dot{V}O_2$). This statement holds true only if the exercise is at a submaximal intensity and $\dot{V}O_2$ is at a physiological steady state. At the onset of submaximal exercise, energy requirements by working muscle increase immediately, however, the aerobic system takes 2-3 min to be fully activated and provide all the necessary ATP. This is illustrated by the rapid, but not immediate, rise in $\dot{V}O_2$ at the onset of exercise or an increase of exercise intensity (Figure 9.1).

During the initial period at the beginning of submaximal exercise, working muscles don't produce sufficient ATP to match the ATP expenditure by the muscle. Consequently, alternate (anaerobic) energy pathways must produce enough ATP during this time to supplement the aerobic system until it becomes fully activated. During this time, PCr hydrolysis and anaerobic glycolysis contribute ATP, but without using oxygen.

However, these anaerobic pathways should not be viewed as producing "free" ATP, free in the sense that oxygen is not needed. After PCr is hydrolyzed to creatine (Cr), the Cr must eventually be synthesized back to PCr, which

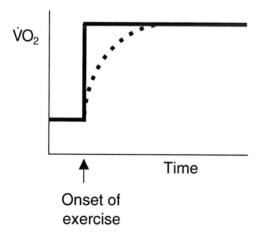

FIGURE 9.1. Representation of submaximal exercise energy expenditure and $\dot{V}O_2$. Energy expenditure is indicated by the solid heavy line and $\dot{V}O_2$ is represented by the dotted line. Note that at the onset of exercise, energy expenditure rises immediately while $\dot{V}O_2$ takes several minutes to achieve steady state.

requires ATP. This is accomplished by the reverse reaction of PCr hydrolysis; the high-energy phosphate of an ATP is transferred to a Cr to resynthesize PCr.

$$PCr + ADP \xleftarrow{\text{creatine kinase}} Cr + ATP$$

Cr moves to the mitochondrial membrane where it is rephosphorylated back to PCr with aerobically produced ATP. Most of this occurs within the first several minutes of exercise recovery, and the aerobic production of ATP used to replenish PCr stores is a primary reason for the large elevation in $\dot{V}O_2$ in the first several minutes following exercise.

In addition, lactate produced in fast-twitch fibers by anaerobic glycolysis is removed by several processes, one of which is oxidation. In this case, lactate is either transported out of the fast-twitch fibers and taken up by neighboring fibers to be oxidized or it can be transported into the blood and taken up and oxidized by distant slow-twitch fibers. In both cases, the lactate is reconverted to pyruvate and then into acetyl Coenzyme A. The acetyl Coenzyme A is oxidized in the mitochondria, which phosphorylates, in the presence of oxygen, new ATP. Approximately 80% of the lactate is removed in this manner during exercise. Thus, although PCr and anaerobic glycolysis produce ATP quickly and without oxygen during exercise, oxygen is required to complete the oxidation of lactate and for replenishing PCr stores during exercise recovery.

This leads to a question: If $\dot{V}O_2$ represents the total energy expenditure during steady-state submaximal exercise, then how might one estimate the contributions of anaerobically produced ATP during the initial minutes of exercise? To answer this question, one needs to recognize that at the onset of exercise, energy expenditure is increased immediately (see Figure 9.1) and as long as the exercise intensity remains constant, energy expenditure remains constant. The initial portion of exercise during which the anaerobic system is supplementing ATP is termed the O_2 *deficit* (Figure 9.2).

After cessation of exercise, $\dot{V}O_2$ doesn't immediately return to resting levels, rather, $\dot{V}O_2$ gradually decreases even though energy demands return to pre-exercise resting levels (Figure 9.3). $\dot{V}O_2$ after exercise remains elevated for a period of time, above what is needed to maintain the resting metabolic rate. The elevated $\dot{V}O_2$ during the exercise recovery is termed *excess postexercise oxygen consumption*, or EPOC, and is the body's attempt to return to homeostasis.

The return of $\dot{V}O_2$ to resting levels is alinear and includes both a rapid and slow component. Causes of EPOC are numerous. A major reason that explains

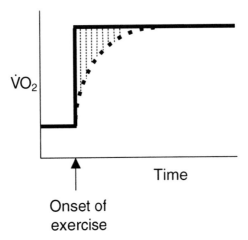

FIGURE 9.2. Representation of the O_2 deficit, which is denoted by the gray area. Energy expenditure is indicated by the solid heavy line and $\dot{V}O_2$ is represented by the dotted line. The O_2 deficit represents the amount of ATP contributed solely from anaerobic sources. This serves as a buffer until the aerobic system can become fully activated and supply all the energy needed for the exercise.

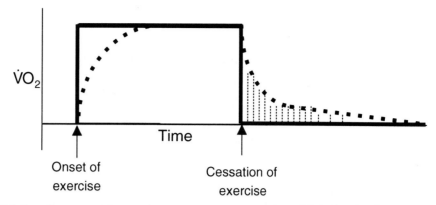

FIGURE 9.3. Excess post-exercise oxygen consumption (EPOC), which is denoted by the shaded area. Energy expenditure is indicated by the solid heavy line and $\dot{V}O_2$ is represented by the dotted line. EPOC represents the excess oxygen utilized during exercise recovery that is above what is needed for resting.

the rapid component is the oxygen being used to produce ATP and replenish depleted PCr stores. Also oxygen is being used during the rapid component to replenish depleted oxygen stores in the myoglobin. The role of myoglobin in muscle is similar to that of hemoglobin in blood. Myoglobin transports O_2 to the mitochondria as well as serving as a storage site, albeit small, for oxygen. Mechanisms of the slow EPOC component are more complex. Included in these mechanisms are elevated body temperature, catecholamines, and replenishment of muscle glycogen.

PURPOSE

The purpose of this lab is to investigate contributions of the different energy systems during exercise through the measurement of $\dot{V}O_2$. In addition, the effects of exercise on $\dot{V}O_2$ during exercise recovery will be studied.

METHOD

In this lab, the changing metabolic rate of a subject going from rest to exercise and back to rest will be followed by the measurement of $\dot{V}O_2$. Prior to data collection, the metabolic measurement cart must be calibrated.

1. Determine resting $\dot{V}O_2$ over a 5-min period in a subject sitting quietly on a chair placed on the treadmill. Before taking any measurements, the subject should have been sitting quietly for at least 10-15 min.

2. Afterwards, remove the chair, and with the subject straddling the treadmill, set the treadmill speed to 135 m · s^{-1} (5 mph). Exercise the subject for 5 min while $\dot{V}O_2$ is being recorded.

3. After exactly 5 min of running, increase the treadmill speed to 175 m · s^{-1} (6.5 mph) and have the subject run an additional 5 min.

4. After the second 5-min bout, stop the treadmill. Return the chair to the treadmill and have the subject sit quietly for 15 min while continuing to measure $\dot{V}O_2$.

1. Graph $\dot{V}O_2$ against time. First, average the last 2 min of the resting $\dot{V}O_2$ data; use this average to plot the 5-min of resting $\dot{V}O_2$. In addition, average the last 2 min of the exercise $\dot{V}O_2$ data for each of the two treadmill speeds. Use the respective averages of the $\dot{V}O_2$ data for *minutes* 3 through 5 and 8 through 10. The purpose of the averaging is to smooth out these data points so that the $\dot{V}O_2$ response can be better visualized. On the graph, denote the rest, exercise, and recovery phases. Draw a line on the graph that indicates the total amount of energy expenditure during each of the two treadmill speeds. *Explain what the steady state $\dot{V}O_2$ for the two running speeds means with regards to the exercise energy expenditure.*

2. Shade the areas on the graph that reflect the amount of aerobically produced ATP. Label these areas. *Explain what the remaining area underneath the line of total energy expenditure represents.* Label the unshaded area appropriately.

3. *Describe under what circumstances $\dot{V}O_2$ does not accurately represent energy expenditure during submaximal exercise. Explain.*

4. *Discuss how the contributions of the energy pathways change during the initial period of exercise.*

5. *Briefly, explain the physiological reasons for EPOC.*

10

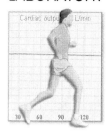

Metabolic Responses to Graded Exercise

LAB DEMONSTRATION

Name_____

As exercise intensity increases, more motor units must be recruited, which necessitates greater ATP production. Furthermore, this changes the contribution of carbohydrates and fats for ATP synthesis. A commonly used tool to study the mixture of fats and carbohydrates by the aerobic system is the non-protein *respiratory exchange ratio* (RER or R), which is the ratio of $\dot{V}CO_2$ production to $\dot{V}O_2$ utilization. (Note: the non-protein RER disregards, though incorrectly, the relatively small contributions of proteins being metabolized for their energy. Actually, proteins contribute about 5% to the total ATP production early during exercise and up to about 15% at the end of prolonged exhaustion exercise.) A ratio of 1.0 indicates that only carbohydrates are being metabolized for energy while a ratio of 0.7 indicates that fats are the only energy substrate. A ratio of 0.83 reflects a 1:1 mixture of fat and carbohydrate metabolism. It is possible for the RER to be greater than 1.0 during very high-intensity exercise, but this will be addressed in a later lab activity. Keep in mind that RER represents the overall fuel mixture by only the aerobic system.

Another physiological measure often used to detect metabolic changes during exercise is measurement of blood lactate concentration ([La]). Lactate is the end product of anaerobic glycolysis and is produced primarily in fast-twitch fibers. During exercise, though, approximately 80% of the lactate is oxidized by slow-twitch muscle for ATP production. However, changes in blood [La] should not be used as a means to quantify anaerobic activity as blood [La] reflects only the net difference between how rapidly La appears and how quickly it is removed.

PURPOSE

The purpose of this laboratory is to investigate the physiological responses to submaximal exercise. In this experiment, a subject will perform several submaximal exercise bouts while $\dot{V}O_2$, blood [La], and RER are being measured.

TABLE 10.1

Speed (m · min⁻¹)	HR (bpm)	VO₂ (mL · kg⁻¹ · min⁻¹)	RER	Blood [lactate] (mmol · L⁻¹)	RPE

METHODS

1. The subject will perform a series of 4-min workbouts of treadmill running (or cycling) that increase in intensity. Each workbout will be separated by approximately 2 min during which time blood will be sampled from a finger stick and analyzed for [La]. The subject will begin running at 120 m · min⁻¹ (4.5 mph), and the treadmill speed will be increased by 15 m · min⁻¹ (~0.5 mph) each workbout until the subject's blood [La] ≥ 5.0 mM (mmol · L⁻¹). Note: If the subject is well trained, he/she should begin running at 160 or 190 m · min⁻¹ (6 or 7 mph).

2. Record the average VO₂ and RER from the last 60 s of each workbout.

3. Record the HR, RPE, and blood [La] at the end of each workbout.

4. In Table 10.1, enter the following data for each treadmill speed: VO₂ (mL · kg⁻¹ · min⁻¹), RER, RPE, HR (bpm), blood [La] (mmol · L⁻¹)

5. Plot graphs of VO₂ and blood [La] against treadmill speed on blank graphs provided below.

QUESTIONS

1. Draw a line of best fit through the VO₂ data. *Describe the relationship of VO₂ and treadmill speed (e.g., linear or curvilinear).*

2. From your graph, predict $\dot{V}O_2$ at a treadmill speed of 168 m · s⁻¹ (6.25 mph). _____ mL · kg⁻¹ · min⁻¹. Mark this on your graph.

3. Describe the effect of running speed on carbohydrate metabolism. Support your answer from the data.

4. Describe the relationship of the lactate response to running speed (e.g., linear or curvilinear).

5. Identify the treadmill speed at which the lactate threshold occurred. _____ m · min⁻¹. Mark this speed on your graph.

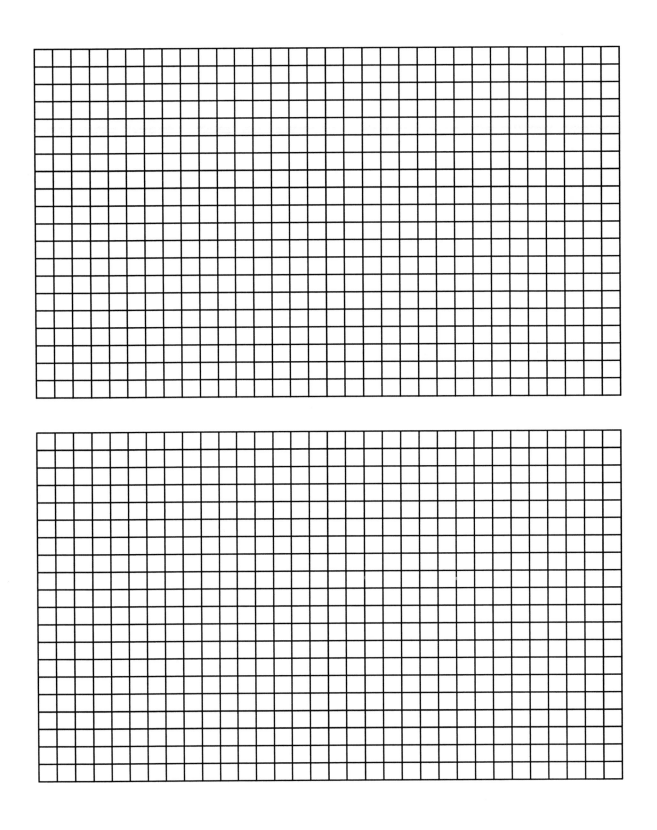

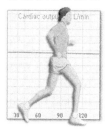

Direct Measurement of Maximal Aerobic Utilization ($\dot{V}O_{2max}$)

LAB DEMONSTRATION

Name_____

Oxygen uptake ($\dot{V}O_2$) is linearly related to workload; as exercise intensity increases, $\dot{V}O_2$ increases proportionally. However, there comes a point at which $\dot{V}O_2$ ceases to rise in spite of any further increase in exercise intensity. The point at which $\dot{V}O_2$ fails to increase any further is referred to as the maximal oxygen uptake ($\dot{V}O_{2max}$) and is considered the benchmark of maximal aerobic power.

$\dot{V}O_{2max}$ assesses the maximal ability of the body to deliver and utilize oxygen and it is related to the ability to perform prolonged exercise. Various physiological factors contribute to the body's ability to transport oxygen, which include:

a) pulmonary ventilation,

b) diffusion of oxygen from the alveoli to blood,

c) cardiac performance,

d) redistribution of blood to working skeletal muscle, and

e) extraction and utilization of oxygen by working skeletal muscle.

Historically, VO_{2max} was thought to be limited by the pumping capacity of the heart. Early studies observed a relationship with heart size and stroke volume (SV) to $\dot{V}O_{2max}$, and that an elevated $\dot{Q}$ was thought to be the critical factor for an improved VO_{2max}. In the late 1960s, a new era began in exercise physiology with the availability of improved techniques to study muscle blood flow and the oxidative enzymes. Subsequent studies sparked a debate as to whether the ability of the mitochondria to utilize oxygen might be the real limitation of $\dot{V}O_{2max}$. There is the potential that oxygen utilization is limited by the Krebs' cycle because of its rate-limiting enzymes. Opinions were to swing back, however, in the 1980s in support of the central limitation argument as more sophisticated techniques for studying blood flow concluded that the more oxygen available to the muscle, the higher the oxygen uptake. Although still slightly controversial, the central limitation argument is held by most researchers today.

Although there are many factors that affect oxygen delivery and $\dot{V}O_{2max}$, the two factors that influence $\dot{V}O_2$ are cardiac output ($\dot{Q}$), and the extraction of oxygen from the blood (a-v O_2 diff). Using the Fick equation, the product of these two factors determines $\dot{V}O_{2max}$.

$$\dot{V}O_{2max} = Q_{max} \times \text{maximal a-v } O_2 \text{ diff}$$

By far, the best method to assess aerobic capacity is to directly measure $\dot{V}O_{2max}$ in the laboratory. Various protocols can be used and require the subject to exercise to exhaustion. However, treadmill tests generally give higher values than cycle protocols. This may be due to greater muscle mass being utilized during running activity than is used during cycling, or because most individuals are less accustomed to cycling than they are with walking or running.

The accuracy of a $\dot{V}O_{2max}$ test can be optimized by achievement of several criteria: (1) a plateau of $\dot{V}O_2$ with an increase in workload (although a plateau often not achieved with many subjects); (2) an RER that exceeds 1.10; (3) a plateau of heart rate and being within ±15 bpm of the subject's predicted HR_{max}; (4) a blood lactate concentration greater than 8 mM; and (5) volitional exhaustion of the subject. Thus, each test should be evaluated to whether or not a true $\dot{V}O_{2max}$ was achieved.

PURPOSE

The purpose of this laboratory is to observe a maximal treadmill $\dot{V}O_{2max}$ test.

METHODS

Prior to administering a maximal exercise test, the subject should complete a *Physical Activity Readiness Questionnaire* (PAR-Q) (Appendix G) to determine whether he/she has any pre-existing medical conditions that would preclude him/her from the test. A variety of exercise protocols can be used, but the highest $\dot{V}O_{2max}$ are obtained during protocols in which the subject is fatigued within 4-10 min. In this protocol, the subject will warm up for ~5 min at a submaximal speed. After a brief rest, the subject will run at a constant speed although the treadmill grade will be increased 2% every minute until he/she reaches exhaustion. This protocol would be described as a maximal, continuous incremental treadmill test. Alternatively, a cycle ergometer could be used. Briefly, the subject would begin pedaling at 50 W. Every minute, additional resistance should be applied to increase the power output in 25 W increments until the subject reaches exhaustion. Afterwards, perform the requested data plots and answer the italicized questions.

QUESTIONS

1. Consider the highest $\dot{V}O_2$ (mL $\cdot$ kg^{-1} $\cdot$ min^{-1}) for a 20-s period (or a 30-s period depending upon how the metabolic cart reports the data) as $\dot{V}O_{2max}$. *Record this value:* _____ mL $\cdot$ kg^{-1} $\cdot$ min^{-1}

2. *Discuss whether the subject achieved a "true" $\dot{V}O_{2max}$ during the treadmill test.*

3. *Evaluate the measured $\dot{V}O_{2max}$ using published norms (Appendix I).*

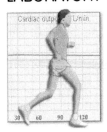

Field Tests for Estimating Maximal Aerobic Utilization ($\dot{V}O_{2max}$)

STUDENT ACTIVITY INVESTIGATION   Name_____

While laboratory testing using indirect calorimetry is the most accurate method to determine $\dot{V}O_{2max}$, the procedure is expensive and time-consuming. Field tests were developed in order to test large numbers of subjects more quickly and easily and are based on their correlation with laboratory tests. Cooper's 12-minute and 1.5-mile runs are two of the most widely known and used field tests. However, these maximal tests require a highly motivated subject exercising to voluntary exhaustion in order to optimize the test's predication ability. Not all individuals are motivated to perform a maximal test, and certain contraindications prohibit maximal testing of all individuals. Consequently, tests to estimate $\dot{V}O_{2max}$ were devised based on the HR response at a submaximal workload. These methods commonly utilize bench stepping, cycle ergometry, and walking/running protocols and are able to quickly test large groups of individuals. Some of the more well-known prediction tests include the Harvard Step Test and the Åstrand-Rhyming nomogram.

PURPOSE

The purpose of this laboratory is to estimate your own $\dot{V}O_{2max}$ using two different submaximal protocols. These protocols will be performed on a running track or some other place that is level and in which the distance can be accurately measured at 1 mile.

METHODS

Before leaving the lab, each person should record her/his weight to the nearest 0.1 kg. Each person will jog 1 mile at a constant (steady) pace. Do NOT speed up near the end of the run. Also, males cannot run faster than 8:00 and females cannot run faster than 9:00. Immediately on finishing, record heart rate and finishing time. Convert the finishing time to minutes and fraction of a minute. Use the following equation to estimate $\dot{V}O_{2max}$.

ESTIMATION OF $\dot{V}O_{2MAX}$ FROM 1-MILE JOG[12]

$$\dot{V}O_{2max} \ (mL \cdot kg^{-1} \cdot min^{-1}) = 100.5 + [8.344 \times Sex \ (female=0, \ male=1)]$$
$$- [0.1636 \times Weight \ (kg)] - [1.438 \times Time \ (min)] - [0.1928 \times HR \ (bpm)]$$

An alternative to the jogging protocol is a walking protocol. Follow the same guidelines as above, and use the following equation to estimate $\dot{V}O_{2max}$.

ESTIMATION OF $\dot{V}O_{2MAX}$ FROM 1-MILE WALK[22]

$$\dot{V}O_{2max} \ (mL \cdot kg^{-1} \cdot min^{-1}) = 132.853 - [0.0769 \times Weight \ (lb)] - [0.3877 \times$$
$$Age \ (yr)] + [6.3150 \times Sex \ (female=0, \ male=1)] - [3.2649 \times Time \ (min)]$$
$$- [0.1565 \times HR \ (bpm)]$$

SHOW CALCULATIONS

Estimated $\dot{V}O_{2max}$ $(mL \cdot kg^{-1} \cdot min^{-1})$ _____

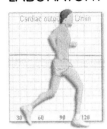

Developing a Submaximal Cycling Protocol to Estimate $\dot{V}O_{2max}$

STUDENT INQUIRY INVESTIGATION

Name_____

In groups of 3-4 students, develop and perform a submaximal, incremental cycling protocol to estimate $\dot{V}O_{2max}$ (mL · kg^{-1} · min^{-1}). Hint: Use the following information, some of which you already know.

- HR is linearly related to workload

- At submaximal intensities, HR takes approximately 3 min to reach steady state

- HR_{max} can be estimated by subtracting age from 220

- $\dot{V}O_2$ (mL · min^{-1}) = 2.0 × Power output (kg · m · min^{-1}) + [3.5 mL · kg^{-1} · min^{-1} × Weight (kg)]

Describe below the steps used to estimate $\dot{V}O_{2max}$. Plot the data points on the attached graph paper.

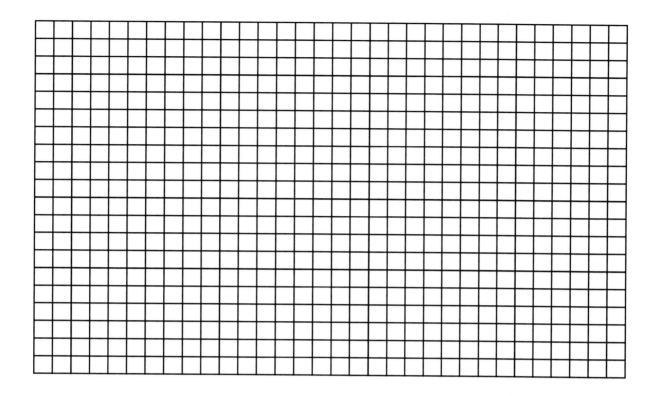

14

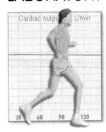

Metabolic Responses to Prolonged Exercise

VIRTUAL LABORATORY INVESTIGATION   Name_____

PURPOSE

During prolonged exercise, a number of changes take place that affect the fuel mixture utilized by working muscle to resynthesize ATP. The primary fuels are fats, from intramuscular and extramuscular sites, and carbohydrates, which include blood glucose and muscle and liver glycogen. In this laboratory, the effects of prolonged exercise on substrate utilization will be investigated.

METHODS

Select the untrained female and run her at 115 m · min^{-1} to volitional exhaustion (60 min). Take measurements of the following variables at 10 min and every 30-min period thereafter. Afterwards, answer the italicized questions.

Pulmonary measures

- $\dot{V}O_2$
- RER

Blood measures

- glucose
- FFA uptake
- glycerol

Sarcoplasmic measures

- glycogen

Blood glucose regulation

- muscle glucose uptake
- liver glycogen
- liver glucose output

CARBOHYDRATE METABOLISM

1. *What is the significance of the RER? What does it represent?* Review the RER data. *Describe the effect of prolonged exercise on RER and what this represents.*

2. *In consideration of the RER response, predict the effect that prolonged exercise had on muscle glycogen stores.* Review the muscle glycogen data to support your answer.

3. Muscle glycogen isn't the only carbohydrate source used during exercise. Review the blood glucose data. *Describe the effect of prolonged exercise on blood glucose concentration. Does the blood glucose response suggest that blood glucose is an important fuel used during the exercise? Explain.*

4. Also, review the blood glucose uptake by muscle. *Explain the response of the blood glucose uptake by muscle in view of the minimal change of blood glucose concentration.*

5. Furthermore, review the liver glucose output. *Provide an explanation for the lack of change in blood glucose concentration when muscle glucose uptake is elevated.*

6. Like muscle, liver also stores carbohydrate as glycogen. *In light of the responses observed above, predict the response of prolonged exercise on liver glycogen stores. Support your response from the data.*

FAT METABOLISM

7. *Knowing what happens to RER during prolonged exercise, predict the response of muscle FFA uptake.* Support your response from the data.

8. Most of the muscle FFA uptake comes from lipolysis of triglycerides in adipocytes. The measurement of blood FFA concentration is not a good marker of lipolysis because blood concentrations reflect only the net change between the rate of appearance into the blood and the rate of disappearance. FFA can appear as well as be removed very quickly from blood, thus a stable blood FFA concentration cannot distinguish whether there is an equal rate of FFA appearance and removal from the blood or there is no movement at all. A better marker of lipolysis is the appearance of glycerol in the bloodstream, as glycerol is removed more slowly. Thus, changes in blood glycerol concentration reflect better any changes in the rate of lipolysis. Review the blood glycerol data. *Explain the significance of the blood glycerol response.*

9. Review the muscle FFA uptake responses. *Discuss the relationship between RER, blood glycerol, and muscle FFA uptake.*

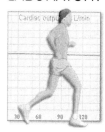

Training Effects on Metabolic Responses to Prolonged Exercise

VIRTUAL LABORATORY INVESTIGATION   Name_____

PURPOSE

Training has profound effects on the body's response to an exercise bout. The alterations in fuels used during prolonged exercise after training can be dramatic. The purpose of this investigation is to investigate these adaptations and to understand the mechanisms responsible for the changes. In this experiment, a sedentary female will perform a prolonged exercise test to exhaustion. After many months of training, she will repeat the test, and because of the training adaptations, will be able to run much longer. One of the purposes of this lab is to determine the reason for this improvement in performance.

METHODS

First, select the sedentary female and take resting measurements of the below variables. Have her perform a prolonged treadmill test for 60 min at 115 m · min^{-1}, 21 °C, and at sea level. Measure these variables every 30 min. Repeat the exercise trial at the same speed and conditions, but instead test the trained female (not the female endurance athlete). After her training, she will now be able to run for 120 min.

The trained subject is the same individual as the sedentary but after having had endurance trained for about a year. Because of her training, her maximal aerobic uptake ($\dot{V}O_{2max}$) increased from 37.2 to 44.5 mL · kg^{-1} · min^{-1}. Often times, exercise intensities are determined relative to one's $\dot{V}O_{2max}$. Note that in this part of the investigation, the two trials are being performed at the same absolute intensities. However, as will be discussed later, during the trained trial the subject will be running at a lower relative intensity, relative to her $\dot{V}O_{2max}$.

Measure the following variables and answer the italicized questions.

Pulmonary measures

- $\dot{V}O_2$
- RER

Blood measures

- glucose
- FFA
- FFA uptake
- glycerol
- catecholamines (epinephrine and norepinephrine)

Blood glucose regulation

- muscle glucose uptake
- liver glycogen
- liver glucose output

Sarcoplasmic measures

- mitochondrial volume (only take resting measurement)
- glycogen

CARBOHYDRATE METABOLISM

1. Review the RER data for both trials. *Describe the effect of training on fat and carbohydrate use during exercise.*

2. The two primary stores of carbohydrate used during exercise are muscle and liver glycogen. *Predict the effect of training on muscle and liver glycogen use.* Confirm your prediction from the muscle and liver glycogen data.

3. *Predict the training response of liver glucose output and muscle glucose uptake.* Confirm your predictions from liver glucose output and muscle glucose uptake responses.

4. *Suggest a benefit of reduced dependence on carbohydrate in the trained state on running endurance.*

FAT METABOLISM

5. Review the plasma glycerol responses of the untrained and trained trials. *Explain the significance of comparison.*

6. Review the muscle FFA uptake of the untrained and trained trials. *Describe the training effect on muscle FFA uptake.*

7. Absolute work during both trials was the same, thus the energy (i.e., ATP) required during each trial was identical. *Considering the training effects on carbohydrate utilization during exercise, rate of lipolysis, and muscle FFA uptake, predict the training effect on fat oxidation. Support your prediction with data from the exercise trials (e.g., RER, muscle FFA uptake).*

MECHANISMS

8. Increased mitochondrial volume results in smaller ADP accumulation in muscle during exercise. ADP accumulation is a major stimulator of glycolysis, thus increases in mitochondrial volume reduce carbohydrate metabolism. *Compare the muscle mitochondrial volume between the untrained and trained state.*

Untrained state _____   Trained state _____   % change _____

9. One of the effects of catecholamines is stimulation of glycogenolysis and glycolysis. Review muscle glycogen utilization of the untrained and trained trials. *Provide an explanation for the training effect on muscle glycogen metabolism. Support your response from the data.*

10. Training is known to increase mitochondrial volume and decrease sympathetic stimulation (catecholamine release) during exercise. *Explain how these two mechanisms serve to increase fat utilization and decrease carbohydrate utilization during submaximal exercise after training.*

LABORATORY **16**

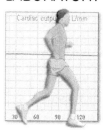

Metabolic Responses to Graded Exercise

VIRTUAL LABORATORY INVESTIGATION   Name_____

PURPOSE

During graded exercise, a number of physiological changes take place that affect the fuel mixture utilized by working muscle to resynthesize ATP. The primary fuels are fats, from intramuscular and extramuscular sites, and carbohydrates, which include blood glucose and muscle glycogen. In this process, considerable lactic acid is produced that the body must remove. This lab will investigate the mechanisms that regulate carbohydrate and fat metabolism and how exercise intensity affects the regulation. Furthermore, the lab will study how the body removes the excess acid produced during high-intensity exercise.

METHODS

Select the untrained male and run him on a graded treadmill protocol that begins at $50 \text{ m} \cdot \text{min}^{-1}$. Treadmill speed should be increased by $25 \text{ m} \cdot \text{min}^{-1}$ every 4 min until reaching volitional exhaustion. Afterwards, answer the italicized questions.

Pulmonary measures

- $\dot{V}O_2$
- RER
- $\dot{V}E$
- $\dot{V}CO_2$

Blood measures

- lactate
- pH
- catecholamines (epinephrine and norepinephrine)

ENERGY EXPENDITURE

1. The measurement of oxygen consumption is used in the laboratory as an indirect measure of energy expenditure. However, the use of oxygen consumption as a measure of energy expenditure is valid only during steady-state exercise. The rate of oxygen utilization ($\dot{V}O_2$) is measured as an absolute value of liters of oxygen per minute ($L \cdot min^{-1}$) or relative to body weight as milliliters of oxygen per kilogram body weight per minute ($mL \cdot kg^{-1} \cdot min^{-1}$). At rest, $\dot{V}O_2$ is ~3.5 $mL \cdot kg^{-1} \cdot min^{-1}$ (~0.25 $L \cdot min^{-1}$). *Predict the effect of exercise intensity on $\dot{V}O_2$. Confirm your prediction from the $\dot{V}O_2$ data.*

2. The maximal rate at which the muscles can consume oxygen is termed $\dot{V}O_{2max}$ (sometimes referred to as $\dot{V}O_{2peak}$). *Describe the relationship of $\dot{V}O_2$ and exercise intensity (i.e., linear or curvilinear). Identify the subject's relative $\dot{V}O_{2max}$ (in $mL \cdot kg^{-1} \cdot min^{-1}$). Use information from Appendix I to evaluate the training status of your subject.*

FUEL UTILIZATION

3. Carbohydrates and fats are the primary fuels used during exercise. The ratio of carbohydrate and fat use changes with intensity. Review the RER data. *Describe and interpret the change in RER with exercise intensity.*

4. Catecholamines are potent stimulators of phosphofructokinase (PFK), the primary rate-limiting enzyme of glycolysis, as well as phosphorylase, which is the enzyme responsible for breaking down glycogen. Review the catecholamine (epinephrine and norepinephrine) data. Glycolysis is the process whereby carbohydrates can be broken down into pyruvate, which is then formed into acetyl Coenzyme A in the mitochondria. In contrast, fatty acids are converted into acetyl Coenzyme A through beta-oxidation. However, at times when energy demands are high, the process of glycolysis is much faster than beta-oxidation. *Hypothesize a physiological mechanism to explain the RER response to graded exercise.*

5. The production of pyruvate is the final step of glycolysis from which there are two primary pathways for pyruvate metabolism. One pathway is for pyruvate to enter the mitochondria and form acetyl Coenzyme A. The other is for pyruvate to remain in the sarcoplasm and form lactate, which then can be transported into the blood. Lactate production occurs when the rate of pyruvate production from glycolysis becomes faster than the mitochondrial oxidation of pyruvate. In addition, as exercise intensity increases, so does the recruitment of fast-twitch muscle fibers, which rely more on glycolysis than oxidative phosphorylation for ATP resynthesis. *Using the above information and knowing the catecholamine response to increasing exercise intensity, predict the blood lactate response to graded exercise. Confirm your prediction from the blood lactate data. Describe the relationship of the blood lactate response to graded exercise (i.e., linear, curvilinear). Afterwards, compare the blood epinephrine and lactate responses. Provide a physiological explanation to explain the close relationship between the appearance of blood lactate and epinephrine.*

6. Lactate threshold is defined as the exercise intensity at which the blood lactate concentration begins an exponential increase over baseline values. *Identify the treadmill speed of the lactate threshold. Also, determine the percent of $\dot{V}O_{2max}$ at which the lactate threshold occurred.*

7. When lactic acid is formed in the body, it quickly dissociates into a negatively charged lactate ion and a positively charged proton (H^+). The H^+ concentration is measured by the pH scale that ranges from 0 to 14 and is inversely related to the concentration. Normal resting blood pH is about 7.4, which is slightly alkaline. *Knowing the large increase in blood lactate accumulation, predict the change in blood pH with increasing exercise intensity.* Confirm your prediction from the blood pH and lactate data. *Describe the relationship between the two variables. Does this relationship support your prediction?*

8. The body attempts to maintain blood pH within a narrow range. The accumulation of acid (i.e., H^+) in the blood is buffered primarily by bicarbonate (HCO_3^-).

$$H^+ + HCO_3^- \longleftrightarrow H_2CO_3 \xleftrightarrow{\text{carbonic anhydrase}} CO_2 + H_2O$$

Thus, the buffering of H+ from lactic acid helps to maintain blood pH and results in the production of CO_2. *Predict the effect of exercise intensity on* $\dot{V}CO_2$. Confirm your prediction from the $\dot{V}CO_2$ responses. *Identify the breakpoint in the* $\dot{V}CO_2$ *data.* Note: unlike the lactate threshold, it will be a subtle breakpoint. Compare the $\dot{V}CO_2$ and blood lactate data. *Explain the significance of the location of the* $\dot{V}CO_2$ *breakpoint. Provide a physiological explanation for the breakpoint.*

9. A stimulator of ventilation is a decrease in blood pH. The H+ stimulate chemoreceptors located in the aortic arch and carotid bodies. Review the pH data. *In view of the pH response, predict the* $\dot{V}E$ *response to graded exercise.* Confirm your prediction from the $\dot{V}E$ data. *Identify the breakpoint in* $\dot{V}E$.

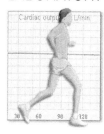

Training Effects on Metabolic Responses to Graded Exercise

VIRTUAL LABORATORY INVESTIGATION   Name_____

METHODS

Select the untrained male and run him on a graded treadmill protocol that begins at 50 m · min⁻¹. Treadmill speed should be increased by 25 m · min⁻¹ every 4 min until reaching volitional exhaustion. Afterwards, repeat the exercise but using the trained male, but begin the exercise test at 100 m · min⁻¹. Afterwards, answer the italicized questions.

Pulmonary measures

- $\dot{V}O_2$
- RER
- $\dot{V}E$
- $\dot{V}CO_2$

Blood measures

- lactate
- pH
- catecholamines (epinephrine and norepinephrine)

ENERGY EXPENDITURE

1. Compare the resting energy expenditure between the two subjects. *Describe the effect of training on resting energy expenditure.*

2. Compare the $\dot{V}O_2$ of both trials. *Describe the effect of training on energy expenditure for comparable submaximal running speeds. Justify the reason for this observation.*

3. Compare the $\dot{V}O_{2max}$ between the two trials. *Calculate the percent increase in $\dot{V}O_{2max}$ that resulted from the endurance-training program.*

FUEL UTILIZATION

4. Review the catecholamine responses for each trial. *Describe the effect of endurance training on the epinephrine and norepinephrine release for comparable submaximal running speeds.*

5. Increases in the mitochondrial volume are directly related to the muscle's ability to oxidize fatty acids. Compare the mitochondrial volume in the subject before and after training. *From the training adaptations observed in catecholamine release and mitochondrial volume, predict the effect these changes have on the mixture of fuels used during exercise. Confirm your prediction by comparing the RER data.*

6. *Knowing the training adaptation on the catecholamine response, predict the blood lactate response to comparable submaximal running speeds between the two trials.* Confirm your prediction by comparing the blood lactate concentrations for each trial.

7. Identify the treadmill speed of the lactate threshold for the two trials. *Explain the potential benefit to performance of the change in the lactate threshold after training.*

8. *Knowing the relationship between blood lactate accumulation and ventilation, predict the effect of endurance training on the ventilatory threshold.* Confirm your prediction by comparing the $\dot{V}E$ responses of the two trials.

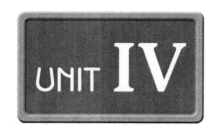

UNIT **IV**

Special Topics

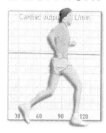

Thermoregulatory Responses to Prolonged Exercise

VIRTUAL LABORATORY INVESTIGATION   Name_____

Humans are only about 25% efficient converting the chemical energy in food to mechanical energy for movement; the remaining energy is lost as heat. In order to ensure that the body temperature remains within a narrow range of 37 to 40 °C (98 to 104 °F), the body regulates body temperature and dissipates extra heat into the environment. Four mechanisms are used to prevent heat buildup.

- *Conduction* — transfer of heat through direct contact,

- *Convection* — transfer of heat through air or liquid as is passes over the body,

- *Radiation* — transfer of heat through electromagnetic waves, and

- *Evaporation* — transfer of heat to convert liquid water to a vapor.

While at rest in moderate ambient conditions, the metabolic rate is low enough so that the magnitude of excess heat is low. The body easily dissipates most of the extra heat through radiation. However, during exercise, the metabolic rate is increased many times and is more than can be dissipated by only radiation. Consequently, during exercise the body relies primarily on evaporation to maintain thermoregulation.

Maintaining thermoregulation while exercising in extreme environmental conditions is difficult. As air temperature increases, the ability to dissipate excess heat via radiation decreases and will even stop if air temperature becomes greater than body temperature. Humidity also affects thermoregulation. The presence of water vapor in air decreases the ability of sweat to evaporate. When the relative humidity (RH) is 100%, the air is saturated with water vapor, which prevents sweat from evaporating. Thus, heat dissipation during exercise on a day with a high air temperature and RH is difficult.

There are two water compartments in the body: the *intracellular fluid* (ICF) and the *extracellular fluid* (ECF) compartments. Approximately 60-65% of the water is in the ICF as it supports cell form and structure as well as providing a medium for metabolism. The ECF is comprised of the interstitial fluid, which surrounds the cells, and the plasma, lymph, and other fluids. Transport of nutrients and waste products occurs via the ECF.

As one sweats, a large portion of water loss is primarily from the ECF, which decreases blood volume and in turn SV. Consequently, HR will increase to maintain cardiac output in order to meet the demands of exercise. Additionally, excessive sweat loss stimulates the release of antidiuretic hormone (ADH) causing the kidneys to reduce urine production and conserve body water.

PURPOSE

The experiment will investigate the physiological responses to thermoregulation and cardiovascular function that occurs during prolonged exercise in the heat.

METHODS

The female endurance athlete will perform a prolonged exercise bout at an air temperature of 21 °C, which will be repeated at the same running speed, but at 33 °C. Select the female endurance athlete and take resting measurements of the below variables. Have her perform a prolonged treadmill test for 180 min at 175 m · min^{-1}, 21 °C, and at sea level. Measure the variables indicated below at 10 min and at every 30 min period. Repeat the exercise trial at the same running speed to exhaustion, but in an air temperature of 33 °C. Afterwards, respond to the italicized questions below.

Thermoregulation measures

- core temperature
- skin temperature
- sweat rate

Cardiovascular measures

- cardiac output ($\dot{Q}$), heart rate (HR), stroke volume (SV)
- BP (systolic, diastolic, MAP)
- total peripheral resistance (TPR)
- muscle blood flow
- splanchnic blood flow
- skin blood flow (SBF)
- hematocrit (Hct)
- plasma volume (PV)

Blood measures

- catecholamines

THERMOREGULATION EFFECTS

1. The core temperature reflects the net difference of heat production and heat dissipation. Review the core temperature responses. *What does core temperature indicate concerning heat production and heat dissipation during prolonged exercise in moderate conditions?*

2. *Since sweat evaporation is a major mechanism to dissipate excess heat during exercise, predict the effect of prolonged exercise on the sweat rate.* Confirm your prediction from the sweat rate data.

3. Note that the subject did not receive any fluids during the exercise. *In light of this and the increased sweat rate, predict the effect of prolonged exercise on plasma volume.* Confirm your prediction from the plasma volume data. *Predict the effect of dehydration on hematocrit; confirm your prediction from the hematocrit data.*

4. *Since blood must be directed to skin to transport metabolic heat produced in the working muscles, predict the effect of prolonged exercise on skin blood flow.* Confirm your prediction from the skin blood flow data.

5. Compare the effects of prolonged exercise in the heat on SV to that of exercise in 21°C. One hypothesis to explain this effect is that increased skin blood flow during exercise will reduce venous return to the heart. *Based on the changes of skin blood flow and plasma volume, predict the effects on stroke volume during exercise.* Confirm your hypothesis from the stroke volume data.

6. A second, recent hypothesis, though, is that the decreased SV is the result of an increased HR[8]. *Recalling that $\dot{Q} = HR \times SV$, and that $\dot{Q}$ changes little during prolonged steady-state exercise, compare the HR responses between the two trials.* Confirm your prediction from the HR response. The phenomenon of the gradual increase in HR over time is often referred to as *cardiovascular drift. Under which condition is cardiovascular drift greatest?*

7. From the above graphs and questions, it can be seen that a variety of physiological responses occurs during exercise in a thermo-neutral environment. These responses serve to prevent an accumulation of core body heat. However, when exercising in a hot environment, the ability to dissipate excess heat may become compromised. To investigate this, exercise the same subject in the 33 °C laboratory temperature and repeat the same measurements as above.

8. Compare the core body temperature data between the two trials. *How might the response of core temperature have affected exercise duration?*

9. *In response to greater change in core body temperature, how might the sweat rate have responded to exercise in the hotter environment?* Confirm your prediction from the sweat rate responses of the two conditions.

10. *In light of the difference in sweat rate between the two conditions, predict the plasma volume changes of the two conditions.* Confirm your prediction by comparing the plasma volume responses of the two conditions.

11. *Considering the greater physiological stress from prolonged exercise in the heat, predict the HR response between the two conditions.* Confirm your predictions by comparing the HR responses of the thermo-neutral and hot environments.

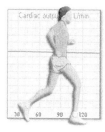

Heat Acclimation on Thermoregulatory Responses to Prolonged Exercise

VIRTUAL LABORATORY INVESTIGATION   Name_____

PURPOSE

An important benefit to regular exercise in the heat is that the body becomes better able to dissipate excess heat generated during exercise. This experiment will investigate the effects of heat acclimatization on thermoregulation, cardio-vascular function, and fuel utilization during prolonged exercise.

METHODS

First, the female endurance athlete who has not acclimated to exercise in heat will perform treadmill running at 175 m · min⁻¹ and at 33 °C to exhaustion without any fluid intake. Repeated the exercise bout using the same subject, but after she trained in the heat for 2-3 weeks. For each trial, take resting measurements for the variables below. During exercise, measure the variables at 10 min and at every 30 min period. Afterwards, respond to the italicized questions.

Thermoregulation measures

- core temperature
- skin temperature
- sweat rate

Cardiovascular measures

- heart rate (HR)
- hematocrit (Hct)
- plasma volume (PV)

Blood measures

- catecholamines

Pulmonary measures

- RER

Sarcoplasmic measures

- glycogen

Additional measures

- Rating of Perceived Exertion (RPE)

THERMOREGULATION EFFECTS

1. The core temperature reflects the net difference of heat production and heat dissipation. Compare the core temperature responses of the two trials. *Describe the effect of heat acclimation on core temperature during prolonged exercise.*

2. *Since sweat evaporation is a major mechanism to dissipate excess heat during exercise, predict the effect of heat acclimation on the sweat rate.* Confirm your prediction from the sweat rates for the two trials.

3. Prolonged exercise in the heat results in cardiovascular drift. This is observed by the gradual increase in HR over time and is related to the degree of hyperthermia. *Recalling the effect of heat acclimation on core temperature, predict the effect of heat acclimation on cardiovascular drift.* Confirm your prediction from the HR responses for the two trials.

4. Consider another mechanism to explain the differences in cardiovascular drift following heat acclimation. Recall that $\dot{Q} = HR \times SV$, that $\dot{Q}$ changes little during prolonged exercise, and that venous return determines SV. *What adaptation must have occurred to the pre-exercise plasma volume that allowed for the smaller cardiovascular drift following adaptation?* Confirm your hypothesis by comparing the pre-exercise PV for the two trials.

5. Review the blood epinephrine (EPI) data for the two trials. *Recalling that EPI stimulates glycogenolysis and glycolysis, predict the effect of heat acclimation on carbohydrate metabolism during prolonged exercise.* Confirm your prediction by comparing the RER and muscle glycogen responses from the two trials.

6. Clearly, heat acclimation has beneficial effects on cardiovascular and metabolic parameters during prolonged exercise in the heat. *How does heat acclimation affect perceived effort and time-to-exhaustion during prolonged exercise?*

LABORATORY **20**

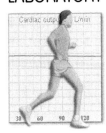

Effects of Altitude on Graded Exercise

VIRTUAL LABORATORY INVESTIGATION   Name_____

PURPOSE

If you have ever attempted to exercise at altitude, you quickly realize it is more difficult than at sea level. This experiment will investigate the effects of running at altitude on cardiovascular and pulmonary functions as well as the lactate response.

METHODS

The trained male athlete will perform two incremental treadmill tests, one at sea level and one at 3000 m (9840 ft). Begin each test at 100 m · min^{-1} and increase the workload 25 W · min^{-1} until he reaches exhaustion. Prior to the test, take resting measurements of the variables below, and at the end of each workload. Afterwards, respond to the italicized questions.

Cardiovascular measures

- cardiac output ($\dot{Q}$)
- heart rate (HR)

Pulmonary measures

- $\dot{V}O_2$
- $\dot{V}O_{2max}$
- $\dot{V}E$

Blood measures

- SaO_2
- epinephrine
- lactate

Sarcoplasmic measures

- Muscle glycogen

Additional measures

- Rating of perceived exertion (RPE)

CARDIOVASCULAR RESPONSE

1. Confirm the added difficulty of running at altitude from the RPE responses.

2. Review the $\dot{V}O_2$ data of the two trials. *Describe the effect of running at altitude on $\dot{V}O_2$ and $\dot{V}O_{2max}$. Calculate the percent change in $\dot{V}O_{2max}$ between the two conditions.*

3. Recall from Fick's Law that $\dot{V}O_{2max}$ is affected by $\dot{Q}$ and the amount of oxygen carried in arterial blood (SaO_2). Thus, either $\dot{Q}$, the amount of oxygen released to muscle, or both, were decreased at altitude. Review the $\dot{Q}$ data of the two trials. *How was $\dot{Q}_{max}$ affected by altitude?*

4. Oxygen pressure is the driving force that moves oxygen from the alveoli into the blood, and at altitude, the oxygen pressure is reduced. The amount of oxygen in arterial blood is measured by the SaO_2, which is the percentage of hemoglobin that is bound with oxygen. *In light of this information and by the lack of changes in $\dot{Q}$, predict the reason why $\dot{V}O_{2max}$ was decreased at altitude.* Confirm your hypothesis from the SaO_2 responses.

5. *Since SaO_2 is decreased at altitude and $\dot{Q}$ is little affected, predict the effect of running at altitude on HR.* Confirm your prediction from the HR responses of the two trials.

6. Peripheral PO_2 chemoreceptors, located in the carotid bodies and aortic arch, are stimulated when the oxygen pressure in the inspired air and arterial blood is reduced. This, among other things, stimulates ventilation and is called hypoxic drive. *Predict the effect of running at altitude on $\dot{V}E$.* Confirm your hypothesis from the $\dot{V}E$ data.

7. Because of the increased stress of exercising at altitude, catecholamines would be expected to be greater at absolute workloads. Furthermore, recall that catecholamines stimulate carbohydrate metabolism. Review the blood epinephrine responses of the two trials. *In light of the above, predict the effect of running at altitude on blood lactate response.* Confirm your prediction from the blood lactate data of the two trials.

8. *In addition, predict the effect that running at altitude had on RER.* Confirm your prediction by comparing RER responses from the two trials.

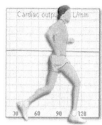

21

Effects of Fluids and Carbohydrate Feeding During Prolonged Exercise

VIRTUAL LABORATORY INVESTIGATION   Name_____

PURPOSE

Prolonged exercise, particularly in a hot environment, stresses a number of physiological systems. Dehydration and carbohydrate depletion occur over time and will adversely affect endurance performance. Fluid and carbohydrate replacement are essential to diminishing fatigue. The purpose of this investigation is to study the effects of a sports drink that contains carbohydrate on thermoregulation, cardiovascular functioning, fuel utilization, and endurance performance.

METHODS

The non-acclimated female endurance athlete will perform two trials in the heat. First, the female endurance athlete performs treadmill running at 175 m · min^{-1} and at an air temperature of 33 °C to exhaustion without any fluid intake. Repeat the exercise bout using the same subject, but for this trial, she will drink 1 L of *Virtual-ade* (a sports drink that contains 6% carbohydrate and electrolytes) that will be consumed in regular intervals during the exercise. Take resting measurements of the following variables as well as at 10 min and at every 30 min interval during exercise. Afterwards, answer the following italicized questions.

Cardiovascular measures

- heart rate (HR)
- cardiac output ($\dot{Q}$)
- stroke volume (SV)

Pulmonary measures

- RER

Thermoregulation measures

- core temperature
- sweat rate
- skin blood flow

Blood glucose regulation

- Blood glucose
- Muscle glucose uptake

Sarcoplasmic meaures

- Muscle glycogen

Additional measures

- Rating of perceived exertion (RPE)

THERMOREGULATION

1. *Predict the effect of fluid intake on core temperature.* Confirm your hypothesis by comparing core temperature of the two trials.

2. The primary heat-loss mechanism during exercise is sweat evaporation. As a consequence of the fluid intake during exercise, heat loss must have been greater in the sports-drink trial. *Therefore, predict the effects of fluid intake on sweat rate.* Confirm your prediction from the sweat rate responses.

3. An additional heat-loss mechanism is radiation from the skin. Blood that circulated through working muscles, where most of the heat is generated, carries excess heat to the skin. *Considering the beneficial effect that fluid intake had on core temperature, predict the effect of the sports-drink trial on skin blood flow.* Confirm your predictions by observations from the skin blood flow data.

4. Dehydration associated with prolonged exercise in heat also affects cardio-vascular function. Observe the HR data from the no-fluid trial. Notice the pronounced HR drift. Fluid intake during prolonged exercise diminishes the HR drift. Fluid intake moderates the increased core temperature and decreased plasma volume that accompanies dehydration and reduces cardiovascular stress. To confirm this effect, on the HR plot, compare the HR responses between the two trials.

5. *In light of the difference in skin blood flow between the two trials, predict the effect that fluid intake had on $\dot{Q}$.* Confirm your prediction by comparing the $\dot{Q}$ responses of the two trials.

6. *Recalling Fick's Law ($\dot{Q} = HR \times SV$), predict the effect of fluid intake on SV during prolonged exercise.* Confirm your prediction from the SV data.

7. Compare the RER responses of the two trials. *Describe the effect of consuming carbohydrate during exercise on fuel utilization.*

8. There are two carbohydrate sources for working muscle: blood glucose and muscle glycogen. *Considering the effect that carbohydrate feeding during exercise had on fuel utilization, hypothesize how muscle glycogen was affected. Confirm your prediction from the muscle glycogen data. Did this support or refute your hypothesis?*

9. *If it refuted your hypothesis, form an alternate hypothesis to explain the effect that carbohydrate feeding during exercise had on fuel utilization.*

10. Review the blood glucose responses of the two trials. Notice that hypoglycemia near the end of exercise was prevented by the carbohydrate feeding. Moreover, the RER data indicate that there was greater carbohydrate utilization during the sports-drink trial, yet carbohydrate feeding had no effect on muscle glycogen use. *In light of this, predict the effect that carbohydrate feeding had on muscle glucose uptake.* Confirm your prediction by comparing muscle glucose uptake of the two trials.

11. Compare the RPE responses of the two trials. Also, compare the times to exhaustion. *What advice would you give to an athlete who is about to compete in an endurance event concerning fluid and carbohydrate consumption during the race? Justify your explanation.*

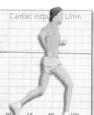

Effects of Diet on Prolonged Exercise

VIRTUAL LABORATORY INVESTIGATION   Name_____

PURPOSE

Diet composition is known to profoundly affect muscle glycogen stores, and glycogen stores affect performance on prolonged exercise. The purpose of this study is to investigate the effects of a high-carbohydrate diet on prolonged exercise.

METHODS

The same subject will be tested on two occasions. Select the female endurance athlete who is has not been heat acclimated and take resting measurements of the below variables. Her diet was previously analyzed and 50% of her total energy intake was from carbohydrates. Have her perform a prolonged treadmill test for 180 min at 175 m · min^{-1}, 21 °C, and at sea level. Measure the variables indicated below at 10 min and at every 30 min period. Repeat the exercise trial at the same running speed to exhaustion, but after having consumed a high-carbohydrate diet (70% of total energy intake) over the previous 3 days. Respond to the italicized questions below.

Pulmonary measures

- RER

Sarcoplasmic measures

- muscle glycogen

Additional measures

- Rating of perceived exertion (RPE)

1. *What effect does diet have on muscle glycogen stores?* Compare the pre-exercise muscle glycogen between the two trials.

2. *In light of the differences in pre-exercise muscle glycogen stores, predict the effect of a high-carbohydrate diet on exercise duration and glycogen depletion.* Confirm your predictions from the muscle glycogen data of the two trials.

3. *Considering the effect of diet on muscle glycogen utilization, predict the effect of diet on exercise RER.* Confirm your prediction from the RER responses.

4. Glycogen depletion is often associated with the onset of fatigue. Predict the effect of a high-carbohydrate diet on RPE during prolonged exercise. Confirm your prediction by comparing the RPE responses of the two trials.

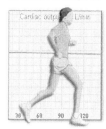

Electromyography

STUDENT ACTIVITY INVESTIGATION   Name_____

Control of skeletal muscle occurs through either a conscious stimulation or a reflex pathway via motoneurons that originate in the brain and spinal cord. Action potentials, electrical "messages," are sent through the efferent neurons and initiate the excitation-contraction process in the muscles.

A single motoneuron may innervate only a few muscle fibers, as can be found in certain eye muscles, but motoneurons usually innervate up to several hundred muscle fibers via branching of the neuron. The motoneuron and all of the muscle fibers that it innervates make up what is called a *motor unit*, and for which a muscle is composed of from a few to several thousand motor units. Muscle fibers contained within a motor unit are usually scattered throughout an area of the muscle rather than being clumped together. Generally, as importance of fine motor control by the muscle increases, the number of fibers in the motor unit decreases. When muscle fibers of a motor unit are innervated, the fibers follow the "all-or-none" law, which means that they generate either maximal tension or nothing. Hence, regulating the number of motor units recruited controls skeletal muscle tension.

Laboratory instruments have been developed to measure and record the electrical activity of muscle. An instrument that records the electrical activity of heart muscle is called an electrocardiogram (ECG or EKG). Similarly, instruments that record the action potentials in skeletal muscle are called an electromyograph (EMG). As the number of motor units recruited increase, so does the electrical activity as well as the size and number of the EMG signals. Consequently, the level of EMG activity reflects the amount of motor unit recruitment and is proportional to the force development. However, EMG activity cannot be used to determine differences of force development between individuals. The amount of electrical activity that is recorded is influenced by the quality of the contact of the electrode with the skin as well as the amount of cutaneous fat, which acts to insulate the electrode from the electrical activity.

PURPOSE

There are two purposes of this lab: One, to investigate the effect of increasing load on the muscle on motor unit recruitment, and two, to study how motor unit recruitment is affected by muscular fatigue. In the first experiment, a subject will perform arm curls with increasing weight while EMG is measured during the concentric and eccentric phases. For the second experiment, the subject will maintain a constant grip on a handgrip dynamometer for as long as possible to examine how fatigue affects EMG activity.

METHODS — EFFECTS OF LOAD ON MOTOR UNIT RECRUITMENT

1. Select three sites on the biceps for electrode placement. Two electrodes will be placed on the belly of the biceps and a third electrode over a bony process around the elbow, which will serve as a ground.

2. Clean the sites by vigorously scrubbing the area for 20-30 s with an alcohol swab. This will leave the area red but removes body oil and dead skin, which is important for obtaining optimal EMG recordings.

3. After the alcohol has dried, firmly place electrodes on the cleaned areas; attach two leads to the electrodes on the muscle and the ground lead to the electrode on the elbow.

4. Start recording EMG as the subject begins to exercise; continue recording throughout the experiment: Using dumbbells of increasing weights, (e.g., 0, 5, 15, 20, 35, and 45 lb), have the subject perform one arm curl with each weight. Instruct the subject to curl in a smooth and continuous manner only to ~45° and all curls should be performed at similar speeds. After completing the flexion movement, he/she should pause for 1-2 s before lowering the weight. The speed of the concentric and eccentric movements should be the same. Upon completing an arm curl, an assistant should replace the dumbbell with one of a greater weight. Be sure that the subject doesn't reach up to grab the weight as this introduces additional EMG tracings. Continue until the subject reaches his/her maximal lift. Record the weights of the dumbbells and the order in which they were lifted. NOTE: Position the electrode leads so that they move as little as possible during the arm curls. Movement of the leads may cause fluctuations of the EMG baseline.

5. Consult your instructor on the specifics for analyzing the data. Determine the integrated EMG (iEMG) voltage of the concentric and eccentric waveforms for each arm curl. Select a representative area of each waveform from which to measure. The length of time for each area to be measured must be identical. Record the data in Table 23.1 below and graph these data against dumbbell weight.

METHODS — EFFECT OF FATIGUE ON MOTOR UNIT RECRUITMENT

6. Prep another subject from your group to measure EMG of the forearm muscles, which flex the wrist and fingers. Two electrodes should be placed on the belly of the forearm flexors and a third electrode for use as a ground.

7. Determine the subject's maximal handgrip strength with a dynamometer. After a brief rest, have the subject perform a constant and continuous grip on the dynamometer at 50% of his/her maximal grip for as long as possible. Record EMG during this time. *NOTE: It is imperative that the subject maintains the grip at precisely 50%, as results will be affected if the tension is allowed to vary.*

TABLE 23.1
Incremental weights and iEMG data.

Weight (include units)	Concentric iEMG (mV)	Eccentric iEMG (mV)

8. Measure the iEMG for the last 2.000 s of each 10-s period. Record the data in Table 23.2 below and graph these data against time.

QUESTIONS

1. *Explain what is represented by an EMG tracing.*

2. *Describe the general relationship between an EMG waveform and skeletal muscle tension.*

TABLE 23.2
Muscular fatigue and motor unit recruitment data.

Time (s)									
iEMG (mV)									

Time (s)									
iEMG (mV)									

Time (s)									
iEMG (mV)									

3. *Explain how skeletal muscle regulates force output. Support your response with your data.*

4. The force-velocity relationship describes how the rate of change in muscle length affects the amount of tension that can be developed. *From Figure 23.1, compare the amount of tension that a muscle fiber develops when allowed to shorten at 0.4 m · s^{-1} to when the fiber is forced to lengthen at 0.4 m · s^{-1} during tension development.*

5. Although the physiological reason for the difference in tension development between concentric and eccentric movements is not well understood, it is clear that such a difference exists. *From your data, compare the concentric and eccentric data. As the force output by the muscle was the same during the concentric and eccentric movements, explain why the number of motor units during the two movements differed.* Hint: Don't consider gravity as the explana-

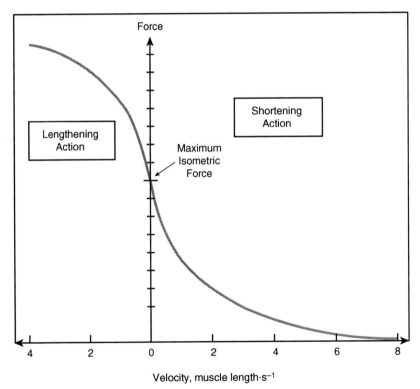

FIGURE 23.1 Force-velocity relationship. Adapted with permission from McArdle, W.D., F.I. Katch, and V.L. Katch. *Essentials of Exercise Physiology.* 2nd ed. Baltimore: Lippincott Williams & Wilkins, 2000, Figure 15.4.

tion for the difference. Rather, return to the force-velocity graph to understand the difference.

6. For the second experiment, recognize that force output by the muscle remained the same—or should have—throughout the trial. *Describe the EMG response over time. Explain the changes in EMG activity. Did the changes in EMG over time suggest that the muscle violated the "all-or-nothing" principle of muscle contraction? Explain.*

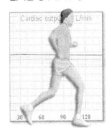

LABORATORY **24**

Body Composition Assessment

STUDENT ACTIVITY INVESTIGATION   Name_____

Most of us are interested in knowing our *ideal body weight*. The first significant attempt at determining ideal weight was made by the Metropolitan Life Insurance Company in 1905. They produced a table of desirable weights by height for adult men and women that was based on compilation of mortality statistics of their policy holders. Met Life continued to revise and update their tables, releasing their latest version in 1983. Unfortunately, their most recent tables were based on information collected in 1959, which led numerous health agencies and experts to criticize the tables for a variety of reasons. Among the criticisms is the fact that the desirable weight values are based on a large, but select, population—Met Life policyholders. Non-Caucasians are underrepresented in these populations and thus, may not typify the average American population. Furthermore, while the tables purport to represent adults from 25 to 59 years of age, one report has suggested that the desirable weight values are too high for younger adults and too low for older adults.

A fundamental problem with the tables was noted in the 1940s by Dr. Albert Behnke, a U.S. Navy physician, who analyzed 25 professional football players. These players ranged in weight from 170 to 260 lb. According to the height-weight tables, 17 of these players were above 15% of their average "weight-for-height," which classified them as too fat for military duty. Yet, a more detailed analysis of these players revealed that 11 of these 17 players actually were below the average percent body fat.

This points to a problem in that the height-weight tables tell us nothing about the amount of fat on our body. Two individuals may both be the same height and weight and classified as normal weight by the height-weight tables. Yet, one of the individuals might be very lean and muscular with little body fat while the other could have less muscle and excessive body fat. To address this issue, researchers developed a model that considers the body to be made up of two components, a *fat component* and a *fat-free component* (i.e., all the tissues and fluids of the body except for fat). A *percent fat* value represents the weight of the fat component divided by the total body weight. For example, a female who weighs 50 kg and has 20% body fat has a body composition of 10 kg of fat and 40 kg of fat-free weight.

Not all of the fat in our body should be considered excess or unneeded. Some fat actually is a necessary body component in such areas as the brain,

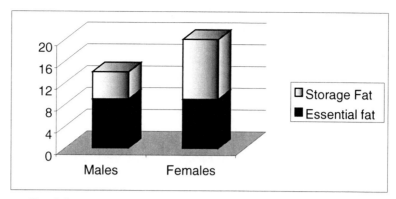

FIGURE 24.1 Total fat composition of a male at 13% and a female at 18% body fat. Most of the difference between males and females can be attributed to the difference in the amount of essential fat.

bone marrow, cell membranes, and heart. This type of fat is termed *essential fat*, and, in males, represents approximately 2-3% of the body weight (Figure 24.1). Females have additional sex-specific, essential fat associated with their reproductive system; the amount of essential fat in females is higher and has been estimated at between 9% and 12% of body weight. While all of us require a certain amount of fat on our body, any additional fat is considered as *storage fat* and simply a reservoir of extra energy. It is the storage fat that we want to reduce when we try to lose weight.

We now return to the original question: What is an appropriate ideal body weight? Body weight alone may not say whether a person is overweight. Rather, body composition provides better information as to appropriateness of weight. For health reasons, males should be no lower than 5% or higher than 20% while females should be at least 15% but no higher than 30%. Generally, suggested ranges for males and females are 10% to 15% and 17% to 22%, respectively (Table 24.1). Most of the difference in the recommended ranges between males and females can be explained by the higher amount of essential fat in females.

For most athletes, however, these ideal ranges are slightly excessive. Male athletes such as wrestlers, endurance runners, and gymnasts perform better at lower ranges. These athletes are often around 5-8%. Wrestlers, basketball players, and football backs tend to be slightly higher, at 7-12%. Likewise, the ideal percent fat for female athletes is lower than for non-athletes. Elite female endurance runners average below 15% while swimmers, sprinters, and gymnasts average 18-20%.

Although there are gradations of obesity, most definitions follow those of the American Dietetic Association; 20% and 30% fat for males and females, respectively. While our bodies require some (essential) fat, too much (storage)

TABLE 24.1
Recommended percent fat ranges for adult females and males.

	Females (%)	Males (%)
Minimum Levels	13 - 17	5
Suggested Range	17 - 22	10 - 15
Overfat	>30	>20

fat increases the risks for a variety of health problems. As percent body fat rises above recommended ranges, health risks increase accordingly.

There are a number of ways to assess body composition. These procedures differ in the time, expense, and expertise required and in the accuracy of the results. All of these procedures are subject to some error and provide only an estimate of the actual percent fat. Errors in a body composition estimate can result from either the actual measurement procedures, the equation selected to calculate percent fat, or both. Most methods were developed from studies on average-weight subjects, which makes estimates of body composition less accurate with very lean or obese individuals. Because of individual deviations from the norms on which the equations were based, accuracy of the percent fat varies from person to person. Variations are associated with stages of growth or aging, exercise history, ethnicity, and gender. For these reasons, even the most accurate procedures of body composition assessment have a standard error of 3-4%. This means that only about two-thirds of all the body composition estimates will be within three percentage points of the actual value while the remaining one third of the estimates are more than three percentage points away. Thus, if body composition were assessed as 18% fat, there is only a 67% chance that the actual percent fat was within 15% to 21%. Consequently, **one should not look at a body composition as a precise measurement, but only as an estimate within a close range**.

The most commonly used methods to estimate body composition are underwater weighing, skinfold measurements, and electrical impedance; they each have advantages and disadvantages. More sophisticated procedures are being used in research settings, but these methods are beyond the scope of this discussion.

UNDERWATER (HYDROSTATIC) WEIGHING

Generally regarded as one of the most accurate methods for body composition assessment, the underwater weighing procedure is based on Archimedes' Principle. In essence, this principle determines the specific gravity of a body and compares it to that of water. Because body fat is less dense than water, it increases one's buoyancy while the fat-free mass, which is more dense than water, makes one sink.

To illustrate this principle, think of two women who both weigh 125 lb. One woman is very lean and muscular and has little body fat while the other has more body fat but less muscle. The fat-free weight of the lean woman constitutes a greater percentage of her weight than that of the overweight woman. The higher fat-free weight and lower fat weight combination of the lean woman increase her body density and make her underwater weight greater.

This procedure requires the subject to perform a maximal exhalation just prior to going underwater. In spite of the maximal exhalation, there remains a small amount of air in the lungs, the residual volume. The increased buoyancy that results from the residual volume must be corrected for in the body density calculations. Residual volume can be measured indirectly in the laboratory using an oxygen dilution technique[39]. Although a simpler method can used to estimate residual volume based on one's vital capacity, this increases the potential error in the body composition estimate. If residual volume is measured rather than estimated, the standard error is approximately 2.5-3.0%.

SKINFOLD (ANTHROPOMETRIC) MEASUREMENT

To find a simpler and less expensive method for determining body composition, scientists investigated the use of anthropometry—the taking of measurements of circumferences and skinfold thickness from different parts of the body. Numerous equations have been developed from anthropometric data to estimate body composition. Among the most commonly employed equations are the *generalized equations* for males and females developed by Jackson and associates in 1978 and 1985, respectively[18,19]. They are termed "generalized" because they have the greatest accuracy for predicting body composition of people within an average range of body fat. Generalized equations tend to be less accurate with younger or older populations as well as the very lean (e.g., athletes) or obese individuals. Other, more appropriate, equations have been developed for special populations that increase the accuracy of anthropometric body composition prediction.

A major source of error in anthropometry lies not with imprecision of the instrument but in the actual taking of the measurements. Making accurate skinfold measurements is more involved than pinching the skin somewhere around a particular area and measuring the thickness. Measurements must be taken at precise sites. Obtaining consistently accurate skinfold measurements requires training and experience. The standard error for this method when performed by a well-trained technician is 3-4%; thus results that approach the precision of underwater weighing can be obtained.

BIOELECTRICAL IMPEDANCE ANALYSIS

The procedure for *bioelectrical impedance analysis* (BIA) involves measurement of the resistance from an extremely low electrical current, which is unable to be felt, as it is passed through the body. The underlying principle of this method is that an electrical current passes more easily through muscle than fat as muscle contains more water and electrolytes for conducting a current. Besides being simple to administer, another advantage of this procedure is that little training or skill are required.

A shortcoming of BIA is that results are sensitive to fluid shifts within the body from exercise as well as the hydration level in which dehydration results in an underestimation of body fat. Likewise, temperature affects the prediction. A warm environment or skin temperature decreases the predicted body fat. Furthermore, this technique tends to overestimate body fat in lean and athletic subjects while underestimating body fat in the obese. While BIA holds promise for making accurate measurements both easily and quickly, this method currently has a standard error of approximately 4%.

PURPOSE

The purpose of the lab is to compare the predictions of body composition as estimated by skinfold measurements and electrical impedance against the estimate by underwater weighing. For best results, subjects should not be measured while in a dehydrated state, following strenuous exercise, or having eaten heavily in the previous 6-8 hours. Work in small groups. Each student should have her/his body composition determined by the three body composition methods used in this lab. Prior to the experiments, your laboratory instructor will demonstrate specifics of the three methods of assessment.

METHODS–UNDERWATER WEIGHING (RECORD DATA ON THE DATA SHEET BELOW)

1. Weigh subject to nearest 0.1 kg.

2. If possible, measure residual volume directly (your instructor will demonstrate the procedure). Otherwise, estimate residual volume from the vital capacity. To do so, measure vital capacity (VC) in a bent-over position using a spirometer. Estimate residual volume (RV) from the VC.

$$RV = VC \times [0.28 \text{ (females) or } 0.24 \text{ (males)}]$$
$$\times \text{ BTPS correction factor (Appendix P)}$$

3. Measure underwater weight from 6-8 trials. Subject must sit quietly in the tank, perform a maximal exhalation and slowly bend over such that the top of the head is completely submerged. Also, encourage the subject to maximally exhale prior to each trial and to remain motionless while underwater.

4. Average the two heaviest underwater weights and record this value as the subject's water weight. Subtract from water weight the weight of the underwater chair. Also, record the water temperature and from this, determine the water density (Appendix Q).

SKINFOLD MEASUREMENTS

1. See Appendix L for guidelines for making skinfold measurements. The equation used in this experiment uses the triceps, suprailiac crest, and abdomen for females and the chest, abdomen, and thigh for males.

2. Record subject's age.

3. Determine and mark the sites for the skinfold measurements.

4. Make at least three measurements; average the measurements and record the average.

BIOELECTRICAL IMPEDANCE ANALYSIS

1. Weigh subject to nearest 0.1 kg and measure height to nearest 0.01 m.

2. Have subject lie flat on table with the right shoe and sock off.

3. Attach two electrodes to the wrist and ankle. One electrode should be placed just above the knuckle of the middle digit and the second electrode between the ulna and radius protuberance on the wrist, and between the fibula and tibia protuberance on the ankle. Attach the red lead closest to the heart—record resistance.

QUESTIONS

1. *From the underwater weighing data, calculate body density* (should be between approximately 1.020 and 1.090). Do not round off this calculation! Note: An estimation of 0.1 L is added to the equation to account for air in the gastrointestinal tract. Note: weight is in kg, RV is in L.

$$D_{body} = \frac{weight_{dry}}{((weight_{dry} - weight_{water}) / D_{water}) - (RV + 0.1)}$$

2. *Use the Siri equation to estimate percent fat from the body density calculated from the underwater weighing.*

Siri equation for estimating percent fat:

$$\% \text{ fat} = (495 / D_{body}) - 450$$

3. *Knowing the total weight of the subject and his/her percent fat, calculate the fat-free weight.*

4. *From the skinfold measurements, estimate body density.*

females: $D_{body} = 1.089733 - (0.0009245 \times sum) + (0.0000025 \times sum^2) - (0.0000979 \times age)$

males: $D_{body} = 1.1093800 - (0.0008267 \times sum) + (0.0000016 \times sum^2) - (0.0002574 \times age)$

5. *Use the Siri equation to estimate percent fat from the body density estimate from the skinfold measurements.*

   Siri equation for estimating percent fat[35]

$$\% \text{ fat} = (495 \, / \, D_{body}) - 450$$

6. *From the bioelectric impedance, estimate fat-free mass (FFM).*

   females:

   $\text{FFM} = [0.475 \times \text{height}^2 \text{ (cm)} \div \text{resistance } (\Omega)] + 0.295 \times \text{weight (kg)} + 5.49$

   males:

   $\text{FFM} = [0.485 \times \text{height}^2 \text{ (cm)} \div \text{resistance } (\Omega)] + 0.338 \times \text{weight (kg)} + 3.52$

7. *From the FFM estimated by bioelectrical impedance, estimate percent fat.*

8. *Calculate the body mass index (BMI).*

$$\text{BMI} = \text{weight (kg)} \div \text{height}^2 \text{ (m}^2)$$

9. *Assess how estimates from skinfold measurement and electrical impedance compared to the estimate by underwater weighing.*

10. *Evaluate the estimate from underwater weighing against normative values (see Appendix M).*

11. *Discuss potential weaknesses of the three methods used to estimate body composition.* Note: This is asking you to assess the methods, not your technique.

12. *Evaluate your technique for each of the three trials. What technique problems increased the potential for error in the estimates of body composition?*

13. *Calculate the amount of weight loss needed to reduce percent fat by 3%.*

    A. Determine the amount of fat-free weight: Multiply the current weight by the fraction of the current percent fat (This calculates the fat weight).

    B. Determine the weight loss needed to reduce percent fat by 3%: Divide the fat-free weight by the fraction of the ideal weight [e.g., if the ideal percent fat is 15%, the fraction of the ideal fat-free weight is (1 − 0.15) or 0.85].

Body Composition Data Sheet

_____
name

Underwater Weighing

dry weight (kg) _____

water weight (kg) _____

chair weight (kg) _____

net wet weight (kg) _____

water density _____

vital capacity (L) _____

BTPS correction factor _____

est. residual volume (L) _____

measured RV (L) _____

Skinfold Measurements

weight (kg) _____

age (yr) _____

females

triceps _____

suprailiac _____

thigh _____

sum _____

males

chest _____

abdomen _____

thigh _____

sum _____

Bioelectrical Impedance Analysis

weight (kg) _____

resistance (Ω) _____

height (m) _____

Body Mass Index

Weight (kg) _____   height (m) _____   BMI _____

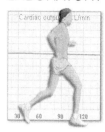

Dietary Analysis

STUDENT ACTIVITY INVESTIGATION   Name_____

PURPOSE

The purpose of this lab is to analyze and evaluate your personal dietary intake.

METHODS

Analyze a representative 3-day diet; select one weekend day and two weekdays. Record everything that was eaten as well as the amounts and type of preparation. It is <u>essential</u> to record accurate measures of the entire food intake including condiments such as salad dressings and butter/margarine added to bread, potatoes, etc. In addition, some mixed foods such as salads, casseroles, may need to be itemized if the specific food item is not listed in the database. Realize that the analysis will be only as good as the accuracy with which you record your food intake.

Using a dietary analysis program, an exercise physiology textbook, or a nutrition book from the library that lists nutritional values of foods, evaluate your diet by recording the following nutritive intakes:

- total energy

- carbohydrate

- fat

- protein

- calcium

- iron

As an alternative, you may choose to use an on-line dietary analysis program. Do an on-line search for a suitable, and free, diet analysis program, or try one of the following links.

- http://www.nat.uiuc.edu/mainnat.html

- http://www.gsu.edu/~wwweat/resources/foodcom.htm

- http://bama.ua.edu/~shancock/NHM201/dietanalysisites.html

DIETARY ANALYSIS

Name_____

Questions

1. *Average the daily energy intake:* _____ kcal · day^{-1}

2. Carbohydrates and proteins have 4 kcal · g^{-1}; fats have 9 kcal · g^{-1}. *Calculate the percentage of energy from:*

   carbohydrates: _____   fats: _____   proteins: _____

3. *Evaluate the above percentages. Does the fat intake exceed the American Heart Association (AHA) guideline?*

4. *Evaluate whether the carbohydrate intake is adequate for an athlete in training. Explain.*

5. *Has your weight remained stable during the past several months? If not, what factors in your diet might be responsible?*

6. *Average the daily protein intake.* _____ g · kg^{-1} · day^{-1}

7. *Evaluate whether your protein intake is adequate for a high-volume weight-lifter or endurance runner. Explain.*

8. What is your RDA percent intake for iron? _____ %.

   If this is low, what dietary changes might you make to increase iron intake/absorption?

9. *What is the percent of RDA for your calcium intake?* _____ %

   Is this adequate? If not, what foods would you eat that could increase your calcium intake?

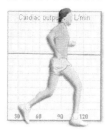

Ergogenic Aid to Anaerobic Performance—Creatine Supplementation

STUDENT ACTIVITY INVESTIGATION

Name_____

Various aids have been and are still being used in the attempt to improve performance. Some clearly benefit performance although many do not. One popular oral supplement, creatine, is being used to improve anaerobic performance and increase muscle mass. However, the literature does not support all claims made about creatine.

Creatine is an amino acid that is manufactured by the body of which about a third of it is bound with phosphate to form phosphocreatine (PCr). Over 90% of all creatine is found in skeletal muscle. Phosphocreatine is highly effective for maintaining ATP concentrations in muscle for short periods of time at the onset of exercise. In human fast-twitch muscle fibers, ATP concentrations decreased only 32-43% from resting levels after electrical stimulation to fatigue while PCr concentrations decreased >90%. As the supply of PCr is limited, depletion of PCr has been implicated as a contributing cause of fatigue in high-intensity exercise.

If PCr depletion in skeletal muscle leads to fatigue during high-intensity exercise, then increasing pre-exercise PCr concentrations may delay the onset of fatigue and improve force maintenance. Following creatine supplementation, though, most studies have not observed improved performance of a single maximal bout. However, many, but not all, studies that used repeated bouts of exercise have reported increased work output after supplementation. Regardless, athletes of various sports have begun using creatine supplementation—which is not on the list of banned substances by either the International Olympic Committee or the N.C.A.A.—as an ergogenic aid to performance.

PURPOSE

This study will investigate the effect of oral creatine supplementation on anaerobic performance. Two sessions will be required to complete the investigation. In the first session (pre-treatment trial), power will be measured for each subject on three different anaerobic tests that will be repeated 1 week later (post-treatment trial). For the 4 d prior to the second session, each subject will consume either 20 g · day^{-1} of creatine monohydrate or a placebo. All subjects in this experiment must be volunteers, have not taken creatine supplements within the previous 8 weeks, and do not have a wheat allergy. Each subject must be unaware of his/her group assignment until after all post-treatment measurements have been completed. First, though, develop with your lab partners hypotheses on the effects of creatine supplementation on maximal anaerobic power and the time-to-fatigue during sprint cycling.

METHODS

1. Prior to lab, purchase the ingredients listed below for the creatine supplement and placebo mixtures. Prepare a sufficient number of creatine and placebo packets for subjects—16 packets per subject (i.e., four packets × 4 d per subject). Note: The placebo contains all-purpose flour, so subjects should be questioned whether they are allergic to wheat flour. If so, they should be excused from the study.

Creatine supplement mixture (enough for about 5 subjects)

In a large bowl, thoroughly mix the following.

- 100 g (1¼ cups) Creatine monohydrate
- 20 packets of non-sweetened flavored Kool-Aid
- 50 g (⅔ cup) granulated sugar
- 100 g (1¼ cups) general-purpose flour

Spoon 1 tablespoon into each envelope.

Placebo mixture (enough for about 5 subjects)

In a large bowl, thoroughly mix the following.

- 20 packets of non-sweetened flavored Kool-Aid
- 50 g (⅔ cup) granulated sugar
- 200 g (2½ cups) general-purpose flour

Spoon 1 tablespoon into each envelope.

Instructions for use

1. First, ask each subject whether he/she has an allergy to wheat flour. If so, the subject must not participate in the study unless the flour is removed from the mixture. Four times daily, subjects should drink 8 oz of water in which one packet was dissolved. If a subject forgets to take a dose, it should be included with the next dosage. Continue the dosage through 4 d.

2. At the first session, perform the following tests in the order indicated. Record results in Tables 26.1 and 26.2 below.

TABLE 26.1
Placebo group results.

Subject	Weight (kg)		Vertical jump (cm)		Margaria power (W)		Cycling test (s)	
	Pre-	Post-	Pre-	Post-	Pre-	Post-	Pre-	Post-
Mean								

- *Vertical jump* (record best of three trials).

- *Margaria stair-climb test* (if timing mats are available). Your instructor will describe the protocol and the site for this test. Briefly, timing mats capable of recording times to the nearest 0.001 s are placed on approximately the fourth and twelfth step. Stepping on the first mat activates the timing mechanism and stepping on the second mat stops the timer. A subject takes a short sprint (about 2 m) to the stairs and climbs the steps two at a time until reaching the second timing mat. The vertical distance that the subject raised his/her body mass divided by the time it took from the first to the second timing mat determines the power. Several trials should be attempted.

- Power (W) = body weight (kg) × vertical distance (m) ÷ time (s)

- *Sprint-cycling fatigue test.* Subjects will perform repeated 20-s cycling bouts until exhaustion. Bouts are to be separated with 40-s rest periods. Use

TABLE 26.2
Creatine group results.

Subject	Weight (kg)		Vertical jump (cm)		Margaria power (W)		Cycling test (s)	
	Pre-	Post-	Pre-	Post-	Pre-	Post-	Pre-	Post-
Mean								

TABLE 26.3
Female Power Setting (W)

Weight Range (lb)	Highly Fit	Moderately Fit	Low Fit
< 110	200	150	100
110-130	250	200	150
130-150	300	250	200
> 150	350	300	250

Tables 26.3 and 26.4 below to estimate an appropriate resistance for the ergometer. The subject should start each bout by trying to reach 100 rpm *as quickly as possible*; apply the resistance when the pedaling frequency reaches 100 rpm. Subject should attempt to maintain 100 rpm during entire bout. When pedaling frequency drops to <90 rpm for 4 consecutive seconds, terminate the test and record total cycling time. Record resistance setting and time to exhaustion. Be sure to offer plenty of encouragement to your subject!

3. Divide subjects into groups based on their performance on the repeated bout cycling test such that the average cycling time for each group is approximately equal. Do not inform subjects of their group assignment. Provide a sufficient number of packets to each subject with instructions for use.

4. At the second session, repeat the tests in an identical manner. Do not provide any encouragement beyond what was given in the pre-treatment test.

QUESTIONS

1. *Explain the rationale for using a placebo group in the experiment.*

2. *Did the placebo group exhibit any change in the post-treatment performance? If so, offer an explanation.*

3. *Do you think that creatine supplementation is an effective ergogenic aid to all types of performance? Explain.*

TABLE 26.4
Male Power Setting (W).

Weight Range (lb)	Highly Fit	Moderately Fit	Low Fit
<170	350	300	250
170-190	350	300	250
190-225	400	350	300
>225	450	400	350

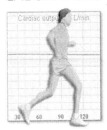

Ergogenic Aid to Aerobic Performance—Caffeine

STUDENT ACTIVITY INVESTIGATION   Name_____

In the late 1970s, two studies came out of David Costill's lab at Ball State University that reported on the benefits of caffeine ingestion to endurance performance[6,17]. The International Olympic Committee (IOC) quickly reacted to these reports and placed caffeine on its list of banned substances in time for the 1980 Games in Los Angeles. Costill and his associates speculated that caffeine increased the rate of fat oxidation, which had a muscle glycogen sparing effect. Numerous studies on caffeine have since followed, but the evidence on caffeine's benefit to performance has been equivocal. Nevertheless, the general consensus is that caffeine does indeed benefit performance. But how caffeine benefits performance remains uncertain. Early studies on caffeine hypothesized that caffeine increased the rate of lipolysis, which made more free fatty acids (FFA) available to the working muscle. With an increased uptake and oxidation of FFA, glycogenolysis was inhibited, thus prolonging the time to depletion. However, caffeine also may increase motoneuronal excitability and increase motor unit recruitment.

PURPOSE

This study will investigate the effects of caffeine on substrate utilization and exercise performance. Two trials, each on separate days, will be required to complete the investigation. Each trial will consist of a 30-min running bout after which the treadmill speed is increased and the subject will run to exhaustion. Because some of the side effects of caffeine ingestion are apparent to a subject, a placebo trial will not be utilized. Instead, subjects will serve as their own control and perform a control and treatment (caffeine) trial. First, though, with your lab partners, develop hypotheses on the effects of caffeine on energy expenditure, heart rate, substrate utilization, perceived exertion (RPE), and time to exhaustion. In addition, prior to the first lab, purchase a package of caffeine tablets (e.g., Vivarin), which are available at most drug and convenience stores. Moreover, all subjects should refrain from caffeine ingestion for 3 d prior to each trial so that all subjects will be caffeine naive (not habituated to caffeine).

METHODS

1. Subjects will perform two trials, each on separate days; be sure that the order of the trials is randomized so that half of the subjects perform the control trial first while the other half performs the caffeine trial first. For the caffeine trial, give subjects the maximal recommended dosage (i.e., 200 mg) 30 min prior to exercising.

2. Calibrate the metabolic measurement cart and lactate analyzer.

3. Although directions are being given for treadmill exercise, a cycle ergometer could also be used. Place and adjust the headgear with the breathing valve on the subject. Adjust the treadmill speed to achieve 70% of the age-predicted maximal HR. This should be accomplished within the first 5-7 min of exercise. Be sure to record all changes made to the treadmill speed and the time they were made, as the identical procedure should be followed for the second trial. Continue running the subject for 45 min. At that point, increase treadmill speed by 50 m · min^{-1} until the subject reaches exhaustion and can no longer continue. Record the finishing time. $\dot{V}O_2$, RER, HR, RPE should be measured at 15, 30, and 45 min. Use 3-min averages (e.g.., minutes 13-15) when taking respiratory measures. Blood lactate concentrations should also be measured at 0, 15, 30, 45, and immediately after exercise. Record the data in Tables 27.1 and 27.2 below.

4. Repeat this trial exactly the way it was performed at the next lab session. Encourage subjects to mimic the exercise and dietary patterns for the 1-2 d prior to the second trial that they did prior to the first trial.

QUESTIONS

1. *Compare the $\dot{V}O_2$ responses of the two trials. Were the responses during the caffeine trial expected? Explain.*

TABLE 27.1
Control trial results (average of all subjects).

Time (min)	$\dot{V}O_2$ (mL · kg^{-1} · min^{-1})	RER	HR (bpm)	Lactate (mmol · L^{-1})	RPE	Time to exhaustion (MM:SS)
0						
15						
30						
45						
Exhaustion						

TABLE 27.2
Caffeine trial results (average of all subjects).

Time (min)	$\dot{V}O_2$ (mL · kg^{-1} · min^{-1})	RER	HR (bpm)	Lactate (mmol · L^{-1})	RPE	Time to exhaustion (MM:SS)
0						
15						
30						
45						
Exhaustion						

2. Compare the HR responses of the two trials. Were the responses during the caffeine trial expected? Explain.

3. Was there a change in substrate utilization either over time or between trials? Support your response using the data.

4. Based on your results, make a conclusion as to whether caffeine is effective as an aid to endurance performance. If you conclude that it does enhance performance, propose a physiological mechanism to explain how it is beneficial.

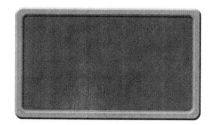

Appendices

Scientific Method

There is a variety of ways that one can obtain knowledge. One can accept as knowledge certain "truths" based on inherited customs or traditions, or one could obtain knowledge from an authority figure. Additionally, one could use deductive reasoning to obtain knowledge or use trial and error. However, knowledge that comes from truths based on traditions or authority figures may not always be correct. Deductive reasoning is based on making assumptions from existing knowledge and has no built-in method to determine the accuracy of those assumptions. Further, the trial-and-error method can be haphazard and unsystematic. The *scientific method* to acquiring knowledge combines important features from the above processes that are generally more reliable for obtaining information. However, the most important aspect that distinguishes the scientific method is that it includes steps to minimize emotions and biases, which can influence conclusions.

The scientific method is an approach to inquiry that follows a general set of orderly and systematic procedures. This means that the researcher progresses through a logical series of steps in order to answer a research question. The scientific method begins with establishing a *research question* that is answerable and narrow in focus; it must not be so broad as to make it impossible to solve. This is arguably the most important component of a research project; the research question is the focus of the project and dictates how the study will be investigated. In addition, one also develops a hypothesis to the research question—an educated guess of the outcome.

Afterwards, the *experimental design* must be developed in such a way as to be sure that the experiment will answer the question. The experimental design is the plan for how the study will be conducted. In an experimental design, the researcher introduces an intervention or treatment (i.e., *independent variable*) while collecting the data on the *dependent variables*. Additionally, a design must include a *control* measurement, which allows the researcher to compare results of the treatment against a group, or trial, in which no treatment was administered. This involves setting conditions so that biases and other confounding factors are minimized in order to isolate the relationships between phenomena. For example, if the research question were to investigate the relationship between perceived effort (RPE) and treadmill running speed, not only does running speed influence perceived effort, but so do fitness level, laboratory temperature, hydration level, and whether the subject recently performed a hard workout. Thus, the investigator must control all other factors that affect perceived effort to be certain that any changes in perceived effort were due to changes only by running speed. In this example, this could be accomplished by having only subjects who were similarly conditioned, being sure that subjects hadn't exercised before coming to the laboratory, testing them at the same time of day, and by adjusting running speed based on a percent of the subject's maximal heart rate.

After *data collection*, results must be *analyzed* to determine whether the independent variable had an effect on any of the dependent variables. In most cases, data were collected on a number of subjects from whom the mean values of the responses are compared. In order to determine whether differences between the means occurred because of the treatment or that differences occurred simply by chance, the means must be statistically compared. Then, results must be *interpreted* and implications of the results examined. If the research hypothesis was supported, interpretation will usually be straightforward, but if the results failed to support the hypothesis, the researcher should offer an explanation. Was there something wrong with the original hypothesis or was the experimental design inappropriate to answer the research question?

The final task of the researcher is to *communicate results* of the investigation. Various forms are used; the most common are to publish results in a scientific journal and present his/her findings at a scientific meeting. Communicating results is essential so that others can build on what already has been established.

Inquiry-Based Research Project Guidelines

Form a group of three or four students—no larger—for your research group. The responsibilities of your group are to:

a) *Develop a focused research question and hypothesis.*

b) *Develop a research experimental design to answer your research question.*

c) *Collect data for the experiment.*

d) *Analyze and interpret the data.*

e) *Develop a conclusion to your research question based on your results.*

f) *Present a 10-12-min presentation on your study results.*

g) *Submit a research paper (typically 5-6 pages in length) on your findings.*

DEVELOPING A RESEARCH QUESTION AND THE EXPERIMENTAL DESIGN

Your group will need to identify a narrow and focused research question that is related in some way to exercise physiology. There are numerous topics from which to choose, but decide on a research question of interest to you. Keep in mind that the question must be within your capabilities, equipment availability, and time constraints. Your research question need not be an original idea nor should it be complex. If you are having problems with selecting a research question, look through your exercise physiology textbook. After finalizing your research question, you'll also need to develop a research hypothesis: What do you predict will be the answer to your research question?

The next step is to determine an appropriate research experimental design, which is the plan for the study to be conducted. The research design should be relatively simple and one that can be completed in the allotted lab sessions. Because of the time constraint, the number of subjects that you test will be relatively small, which may compromise results and make conclusions tentative. You may use group members as subjects, but you'll likely need to recruit outside individuals as well. Five subjects is a typical sample size but the sample size will depend upon time and complexity of the measurements. Depending upon the complexity and length of exercise protocols, some groups may be able to test only three subjects whereas others may be able to test 10 or more subjects.

Perhaps the most important element of an experimental design is control because it allows the researcher to isolate the cause or condition of the treatment. Don't neglect this aspect of your design. There is a variety of ways to include control in a study such as having all subjects perform a pre- and post-treatment measurement. In this design, subjects serve as their own control, and by comparing the pre- and post-treatment measurements, the researcher can determine the effect of the treatment. Furthermore, as subjects sometimes perform better on a subsequent test, the order of the treatment and control trials should be randomized for subjects. Another example is to use separate control and treatment groups. This design requires twice as many subjects as the pre/post treatment design. In addition, it is essential that subjects be randomly assigned to a group to ensure that the groups are equivalent.

COLLECTING AND ANALYZING THE DATA

Your instructor will indicate which equipment is available for your use, although your research question may not require use of your lab facilities to collect your data. Prior to using any equipment, however, you must become thoroughly familiar with its operation. This requires practice time before you begin any data collection! When you actually begin data collection, carefully follow proper laboratory techniques to minimize instrument and human error and to ensure that the data is valid. Should you feel any data from a subject is suspect due to improper techniques, subject noncompliance, etc., repeat the data collection. **Do not submit a paper containing bad data!**

After completion of the data collection, compute means and standard deviations for all your measurements. This is easily accomplished by using Excel, which can also graph your data. Although not required, you may also wish to perform some simple statistics such as t-tests, Chi-squares, or correlations. Keep in mind, though, that a small sample size decreases the confidence one can place in the outcome of a statistical analysis.

After reviewing and analyzing the data, your group should form a conclusion to the research question that is based on your results. A conclusion is the answer to the research question, and as such, must respond directly to it and is supported by your data.

PRESENTING THE RESULTS

If possible, use presentation software (e.g., PowerPoint) for the oral presentations; however, it is not expected be a sophisticated presentation. Plan for your presentation to be 10-12 min in length followed by 5 min of questioning from the class. Keep information on your presentation simple and direct. Additionally, you will need to submit a 5-6-page typewritten paper of the experiment and its results.

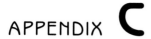

Scientific Paper Guidelines

Organize your paper using the headings below. If warranted, use subheadings within a section to separate divisions of information. It should be written in third person, typed using a 12-point font, double-spaced with 1-in. margins, and all units converted to metric. A paper is graded on a number of factors, but clear writing is important. Although all sections are important to the overall quality of the paper, the *Discussion* section is of greatest importance, as it is your opportunity to demonstrate a comprehensive understanding of the problem.

INTRODUCTION

As the heading suggests, this section introduces the project. It is often written using a "funnel" technique in which the author(s) begins with general statements about the topic that gradually become more focused until finally stating the research question. The research question is usually placed near the end of this section and followed by the research hypothesis. A rationale that explains the reasoning for investigating the research question should also be included in the Introduction. For example, if the topic was on estimating body composition, begin the Introduction by stating:

> *Underwater weighing is considered to be the most accurate of commonly performed body composition assessment procedures. As this procedure requires certain equipment and is time consuming, field-testing large numbers of subjects is not practical. Thus, other methods were developed which take less time and require only minimal equipment to estimate body composition. The purpose of the study is to then compare these methods with underwater weighing. Our hypothesis is that the other methods are not as accurate as underwater weighing for estimating body composition.*

An Introduction such as this begins as general statements but becomes narrower in focus and eventually leads into the statement of the research question. This example, though, should be expanded to state the need to validate the methods, which would provide a clearer rationale for conducting the study.

METHODS

After reading this section, anyone should be able to duplicate your study. Include a description of the subjects (e.g., number, age, weight, gender, fitness level); the experimental procedures and design; and the analysis that was performed (e.g., simple comparison of means, t-test, Chi Square test, correlations).

Avoid providing excessive detail such as how you placed a facemask and nose clip on a subject prior to measuring $\dot{V}O_2$, or all steps that you took to calibrate the metabolic measurement cart. These basic steps are assumed to have occurred. Stating each mundane step in a procedure is unwarranted and merely clutters up the writing. However, include important information such as the number and duration of trials performed or how the data was treated (e.g., recorded only the highest value, averaged the data).

RESULTS

This section only presents and describes the data. It should not contain explanations as to why the data behaved as it did but rather state or describe the effects of the treatment. **Do not report individual data, rather the data should be averaged** and presented in a table or graph. Number the tables and graphs, and be sure to reference and discuss this information somewhere in this section. In addition, all graphs and tables must be appropriately labeled and include units. Although statistical analysis is not required, this information would also be placed in the results section.

DISCUSSION

In this section, the results are interpreted and analyzed. Do your statistics or the data trends support your hypothesis? How solid are the data and do they support your hypothesis? Were there any potential errors that influenced your data? Do not use "human error" to explain poor data; otherwise, you should have repeated the measurement. What physiological principle explains your results? Are there any alternative explanations? How could the experiment be improved? At the end of the Discussion section, state the conclusion to the study. The conclusion must address the research question and be supported by the results. You may end up either supporting or refuting your research hypothesis, or if the results are inconclusive, state the conclusion as such.

REFERENCES

For this project, you are not required to do a literature search of the problem, but if you do use any reference materials, be sure to cite them and include a reference list at the end of the paper. Any information that is used and not commonly known by an exercise physiologist—not discussed in lecture or your text—should be cited and referenced at the end of the paper.

APPENDIX D

Metabolic Calculations

In the exercise physiology laboratory, energy expenditure is determined, indirectly, by the measurement of oxygen utilization. Ultimately, all energy used by the body comes from food transformed by the aerobic energy system, which, as recognized, requires oxygen. Thus, as the amount of ATP used during exercise cannot be measured directly, it can be measured indirectly by the amount of oxygen utilized to synthesize the ATP. Although this doesn't hold true at high exercise intensities, the rate of steady-state oxygen utilization (or oxygen consumption or oxygen uptake), referred to as $\dot{V}O_2$, reflects the total rate of energy expenditure required to perform the exercise. As the exercise intensity changes, so does the amount of energy needed to perform the exercise, and the rate of oxygen required to provide this energy changes in proportion to the energy expenditure (*Equation 1*). Thus, *the rate of oxygen utilization ($\dot{V}O_2$) should be viewed as a measurement of energy expenditure.*

$$\text{Food} + O_2 \rightarrow CO_2 + H_2O + \text{Energy} \qquad (1)$$

The relationship between exercise intensity and energy expenditure is linear, which means that energy expenditure changes in the same proportion with changes in exercise intensity (see Figure D.1). Because this relationship is linear, predicting energy expenditure is simple. All one needs to know to estimate energy expenditure is the exercise intensity and the appropriate metabolic formula.

Although exercise intensity can continue to increase, at some point $\dot{V}O_2$ will cease to rise. This point represents the maximal rate of energy that the aerobic system can provide, and it is referred to as the maximal rate of oxygen

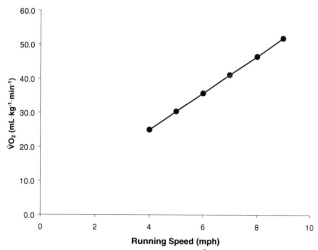

FIGURE D.1. Energy expenditure, as measured by $\dot{V}O_2$ (mL · kg^{-1} · min^{-1}), increases the same proportion with each 1.0 mph increase of running speed.

utilization, or $\dot{V}O_{2max}$. Moreover, the ability to deliver oxygen to working muscles is the limiting factor of $\dot{V}O_{2max}$, thus $\dot{V}O_{2max}$ *can be used as an indicator of cardiovascular fitness.*

The measurement of $\dot{V}O_2$ requires expensive equipment, which is usually not available in health fitness facilities, nor is the measurement of $\dot{V}O_2$ practical for large groups of clients. However, mathematical formulae, correlated to laboratory data, have been developed for estimating $\dot{V}O_2$ in a variety of exercise modes.

When expressing $\dot{V}O_2$ in absolute terms, the units are *liters of oxygen utilization* per *minute* (L · min⁻¹), although $\dot{V}O_2$ is expressed most often relative to body weight, as *milliliters of oxygen utilization* per *kilogram of body weight* per *minute* (mL · kg⁻¹ · min⁻¹). A 50-kg female used oxygen at the rate of approximately 1.5 L · min⁻¹ while running at 5 mph whereas a 100-kg male used oxygen at about twice that rate, 3.0 L · min⁻¹. However, if $\dot{V}O_2$ were expressed relative to body weight, $\dot{V}O_2$ for both individuals would be around 30 mL · kg⁻¹ · min⁻¹. *Equations 2* and *3* show the conversions between absolute and relative expressions of $\dot{V}O_2$, and Table D.1 visualizes this concept for our two individuals running at different speeds.

$$\dot{V}O_2 \text{ (mL · kg}^{-1} \text{ · min}^{-1}) =$$
$$\dot{V}O_2 \text{ (L · min}^{-1}) \div \text{Body weight (kg)} \times 1000 \text{ mL · L}^{-1} \qquad (2)$$

$$\dot{V}O_2 \text{ (L · min}^{-1}) =$$
$$\dot{V}O_2 \text{ (mL · kg}^{-1} \text{ · min}^{-1}) \times \text{Body weight (kg)} \times 0.001 \text{ L · mL}^{-1} \qquad (3)$$

METABOLIC EQUIVALENTS (METs)

Besides $\dot{V}O_2$, energy expenditure is expressed in other ways. One expression commonly used by clinicians is *metabolic equivalents* (METs), which is based on the resting metabolic rate or the rate of oxygen required to maintain functioning of the various physiological systems such as the cardiorespiratory, renal, and nervous systems. On average, $\dot{V}O_2$ in resting individuals is 3.5 mL · kg⁻¹ · min⁻¹; thus, one MET equals the average resting $\dot{V}O_2$. As an example, an individual jogging at 4 mph who is utilizing oxygen at the rate of 25 mL · kg⁻¹ ·

TABLE D.1
$\dot{V}O_2$ expressed in absolute and relative terms at various running speeds.

Running speed (m · min⁻¹)	$\dot{V}O_2$ (L · min⁻¹)		$\dot{V}O_2$ (mL · kg⁻¹ · min⁻¹)
	50-kg female	100-kg male	Both individuals
107	1.25	2.50	25.0
134	1.52	2.77	30.3
161	1.78	3.57	35.7
188	2.05	4.11	41.1
214	2.32	4.64	46.4

min^{-1} could also be described as exercising at about 7 METs [25 mL · kg^{-1} · min^{-1} ÷ 3.5 (mL · kg^{-1} · min^{-1})/MET], or 7 times the resting metabolic rate (*Equation 4*).

$$\text{METs} = \dot{V}O_2 \text{ (mL} \cdot \text{kg}^{-1} \cdot \text{min}^{-1}) \div 3.5 \text{ (mL} \cdot \text{kg}^{-1} \cdot \text{min}^{-1}) / \text{MET} \qquad (4)$$

NET AND GROSS OXYGEN UTILIZATION

Energy expended during exercise is also described in terms of net or gross $\dot{V}O_2$. Gross $\dot{V}O_2$ is simply the total rate at which oxygen is being utilized. Net $\dot{V}O_2$, though, is the gross $\dot{V}O_2$ minus the energy being expended for the resting metabolic rate, which is 3.5 mL · kg^{-1} · min^{-1}. Like one's paycheck, the net, or "take-home" pay, is the gross salary minus all deductibles such as taxes, retirement, and other benefits. All ACSM metabolic formulae were developed to calculate the gross $\dot{V}O_2$; so, *subtracting 3.5 mL · kg^{-1} · min^{-1} from the gross $\dot{V}O_2$ provides the net $\dot{V}O_2$.*

KILOCALORIE

Energy is also commonly expressed using kilocalories, or Calorie (with a capital C). Units of energy can be converted between various expressions such as converting energy expressed as $\dot{V}O_2$ into kilocalories. The use of 5 L of oxygen results in the expenditure of approximately 5 kcal of energy (*Equation 5*).

$$\text{Rate of energy expenditure (kcal} \cdot \text{min}^{-1}) = \qquad (5)$$
$$\dot{V}O_2 \text{ (L} \cdot \text{min}^{-1}) \times 5 \text{ kcal} \cdot \text{L}^{-1}$$

Furthermore, the *total* energy expenditure of an exercise—as opposed to the *rate* of energy expenditure—can be calculated by multiplying the rate of energy expenditure by the exercise duration (*Equation 6*).

$$\text{Total energy expenditure (kcal)} = \qquad (6)$$
$$\text{Energy rate (kcal} \cdot \text{min}^{-1}) \times \text{Exercise duration (min)}$$

In addition, the amount of fat utilized during the exercise period can be estimated from the total energy expenditure. One pound of fat is equivalent to approximately 3500 kcal, thus, one would need to expend an extra 3500 kcal through exercise, eat 3500 fewer kilocalories of food, or a combination of the two in order to lose 1 lb of fat (*Equation 7*).

$$\text{Fat loss (lb)} = \text{Total energy expenditure (kcal)} \div 3500 \text{ (kcal} \cdot \text{lb}^{-1}) \qquad (7)$$

CONVERTING UNITS OF POWER, OR WORK RATE, FROM KG-M · MIN⁻¹ TO WATTS (W)

Watts (W) is a unit of power, or work rate, that describes how rapidly a force is applied and is typically used to express power with arm- or leg-cycle ergometers.

TABLE D.2

ACSM metabolic formulas for estimating relative $\dot{V}O_2$ (mL · kg^{-1} · min^{-1}) during various exercise modes.

Walking	= [0.1 × Speed (m · min^{-1})] + [1.8 × Speed (m · min^{-1}) × Grade (% expressed as fraction) + 3.5 mL · kg^{-1} · min^{-1}
Treadmill and Outdoor Running	= [0.2 × Speed (m · min^{-1})] + [0.9 × Speed (m · min^{-1}) × Grade (% grade expressed as fraction) + 3.5 mL · kg^{-1} · min^{-1}
Leg Ergometry	= [10.8 × Power (W) ÷ Body weight (kg)] + 7 mL · kg^{-1} · min^{-1}
Arm Ergometry	= [18 × Power (W) ÷ Body weight (kg)] + 3.5 mL · kg^{-1} · min^{-1}
Stepping	= [0.2 × Stepping rate (steps · min^{-1})] + [1.33 × 1.8 × Stepping rate (steps · min^{-1}) × Step height (m)] + 3.5 mL · kg^{-1} · min^{-1}

Adapted with permission from *ACSM's Guidelines for Exercise Testing and Prescription*. 6th ed. Baltimore: Lippincott Williams & Wilkins, 2000, Table D-1.

To calculate power, the resistance and cycling speed must be known. The resistance is usually expressed as kiloponds or kilograms, and cycling speed is the product of the pedaling revolution and the flywheel circumference of the cycle ergometer. On the Monark leg-cycle ergometers, the flywheel circumference is 6.0 m.

Example: Calculate the work rate (W), or power, of a client, pedaling at 60 rpm at 2.0 kp of resistance.

1. 2.0 kp = 2.0 kg

2. Cycling speed = 50 rpm × 6.0 m · rev^{-1} = 300 m · min^{-1}

3. Work rate (kg-m · min^{-1}) = 2.0 kg × 300 m · min^{-1} = 600 kg-m · min^{-1}

4. 1 W = 6 kg-m · min^{-1}, so divide kg-m · min^{-1} by 6 to convert power to Watts

5. Work rate (W) = 600 kg-m · min^{-1} ÷ 6 W/(kg-m · min^{-1}) = 100 W mL · kg^{-1} · min^{-1}

ALGEBRAIC REMINDERS

NOTE: *Calculators are programmed to observe the mathematical order; thus, in most equations used in the metabolic formulae, one needs only to enter the appropriate number followed by the mathematical function in the order presented in the equation to obtain the correct solution.*

- There is a mathematical order for performing various functions. Perform exponential (e.g., 24^2) first, followed by multiplications and divisions, and additions and subtractions last.

     Example: $\dot{V}O_2$ (mL · kg^{-1} · min^{-1}) = [0.1 × 88.4 m · min^{-1}] + [1.8 × 88.4 m · min^{-1} × 0.04] + 3.5 mL · kg^{-1} · min^{-1}

     - To solve, first multiply the 0.1 and 88.44, and then the 1.8 and 88.4.
     - Add the two products to 3.5

- There will be times when the unknown value to solve is not separated from the known values (e.g., 25.5 L · min^{-1} = 89 beats · min^{-1} × Stroke volume (mL · beat^{-1}). In these situations, the known values must be placed on the other side of the equal sign in order to solve for the unknown.

  Example: 17.5 mL · kg^{-1} · min^{-1} = [0.2 × Stepping rate (steps · min^{-1})] + [1.33 × 1.8 × Stepping rate (steps) × 0.127 m] + 3.5 mL · kg^{-1} · min^{-1}

  - To solve for the *Stepping rate*, first move the 3.5 mL · kg^{-1} · min^{-1} to the other side of the equation. In doing so, the addition sign becomes a subtraction sign.

    17.5 mL · kg^{-1} · min^{-1} - 3.5 mL · kg^{-1} · min^{-1} = [0.2 × Stepping rate (steps · min^{-1})] + [1.33 × 1.8 × Stepping rate (steps · min^{-1}) × 0.127 m]

  - Next, recognize that the two following equations are equal. In the first equation, *Stepping rate* was used in both brackets, so the second equation was rearranged so that it is used only once.

    [0.2 × Stepping rate (steps · min^{-1})] + [1.33 × 1.8 × Stepping rate (steps · min^{-1}) × 0.127 m]

    Stepping rate (steps · min^{-1}) × [(0.2) + (1.33 × 1.8 × 0.127)]

  - Lastly, the bracketed numbers from the second equation immediately above were moved to the other side which leaves all the known values on the other side of the equation from *Stepping rate*. However, when the bracketed numbers were switched to the other side, instead of being used to multiply, they changed to divide.

    [17.5 mL · kg^{-1} · min^{-1} - 3.5 mL · kg^{-1} · min^{-1}] ÷ [(0.2) + (1.33 × 1.8 × 0.127)] = Stepping rate (steps · min^{-1})

  - Remember, first move all added and subtracted numbers <u>that are not being multiplied or divided by other numbers</u> to one side. In doing so, the sign is changed from addition to subtraction or vice versa.

  - Whenever a number that is being divided or multiplied is moved to the other side, its mathematical function is also changed. Numbers being multiplied are changed to division and vice versa.

Metabolic Problems

Use the metabolic formulae from Appendix D. Solutions to the problems can be found in Appendix F.

1. Calculate the power (W) output of cycling at 60 rpm with 2.0 kg of resistance.

2. Convert the $\dot{V}O_2$ of a 69-kg client from 2.67 $L \cdot min^{-1}$ to $mL \cdot kg^{-1} \cdot min^{-1}$.

3. Convert the $\dot{V}O_2$ of a 43.3-kg client from 29.6 $mL \cdot kg^{-1} \cdot min^{-1}$ to $L \cdot min^{-1}$.

4. Calculate the METs from a client exercising at 34.1 $mL \cdot kg^{-1} \cdot min^{-1}$.

5. Calculate the relative $\dot{V}O_2$ of a client exercising at 6.5 METs.

6. Calculate the absolute $\dot{V}O_2$ of a 43.9-kg client exercising at 25.1 $mL \cdot kg^{-1} \cdot min^{-1}$.

7. Calculate the energy expenditure ($kcal \cdot min^{-1}$) of a client exercising at a $\dot{V}O_2$ of 3.5 $L \cdot min^{-1}$.

8. Calculate the absolute $\dot{V}O_2$ of a client exercising at 7.3 $kcal \cdot min^{-1}$.

9. Calculate the total energy expenditure (kcal) of a client who exercised for 25 min at 11.2 $kcal \cdot min^{-1}$.

10. Calculate the length of the session of a client who exercised at a rate of 5.4 $kcal \cdot min^{-1}$ and expended 245 kcal.

11. Calculate the fat loss (lb) of a client over a 2-week period who expended an extra 544 kcal each of 7 days through exercise. Assume there was no change in diet intake.

12. Calculate the length of time required for a client to lose 5 lb who has increased her daily exercise by 500 kcal and decreased her dietary intake by 300 kcal.

13. Calculate the relative $\dot{V}O_2$ from walking on a treadmill at 3.3 mph with a 4% grade.

14. Calculate the relative $\dot{V}O_2$ of a 124-lb female who used a Monark leg ergometer at 70 rpm with 1.5 kg of resistance.

15. Calculate the relative $\dot{V}O_2$ of a 196-lb male stepping on a 9-in bench at 30 steps $\cdot min^{-1}$.

16. A 122-lb female is walking on a treadmill at 2.8 mph at 2% grade for 30 min. Estimate the
    a. relative $\dot{V}O_2$
    b. METs
    c. total energy expenditure (kcal)

17. A 52-kg client is cycling at 70 rpm on a Monark ergometer with a force of 1.5 kp. Determine how many 30-min sessions of this he would need to perform in order to lose 8 lb of fat.

18. A 181-lb woman is walking on a treadmill at 2.2 mph at a 5% grade. Calculate her

    a. gross absolute $\dot{V}O_2$

    b. net relative $\dot{V}O_2$

    c. energy expenditure in kcal · min^{-1}

19. Calculate the stepping rate on a 6-in. step of a 72-kg client whom you wish to exercise at 5 METs.

20. A 151-lb client wants to lose 15 lb of fat over the next 26 weeks. Assuming she will not change her dietary intake, calculate how long would each daily run need to be if she runs at 5.0 mph on a level treadmill.

21. Calculate the resistance on a Monark leg-cycle ergometer for a 230-lb client to cycle at 50 rpm at an intensity of 5 METs.

22. Predict the number of weeks required for a 185-lb client to lose 20 lb of fat who will run for 45 min at a $\dot{V}O_2$ of 37.5 mL · kg^{-1} · min^{-1} three times weekly. Assume no change in his dietary intake.

Metabolic Problem Solutions

1. *Calculate the power (W) output of cycling at 60 rpm with 2.0 kg of resistance.*
   a. flywheel circumference = 6 m
   b. 60 rpm $\times$ 6 m $\cdot$ rev^{-1} $\times$ 2.0 kg = 720 kg-m $\cdot$ min^{-1}
   c. 720 kg-m $\cdot$ min^{-1} $\div$ 6 (kg-m $\cdot$ min^{-1})/W = **120 W**

2. *Convert the $\dot{V}O_2$ of a 69-kg client from 2.67 mL $\cdot$ min^{-1} to mL $\cdot$ kg^{-1} $\cdot$ min^{-1}.*
   a. 2.67 L $\cdot$ min^{-1} $\times$ 1000 mL $\cdot$ L^{-1} = 2670 mL $\cdot$ min^{-1}
   b. 2670 mL $\cdot$ min^{-1} $\div$ 69 kg = **38.7 mL $\cdot$ kg^{-1} $\cdot$ min^{-1}**

3. *Convert the $\dot{V}O_2$ of a 43.3-kg client from 29.6 mL $\cdot$ kg^{-1} $\cdot$ min^{-1} to L $\cdot$ min^{-1}.*
   a. 43.4 kg $\times$ 29.6 mL $\cdot$ kg^{-1} $\cdot$ min^{-1} = 1285 mL $\cdot$ min^{-1}
   b. 1285 mL $\cdot$ min^{-1} $\div$ 1000 mL $\cdot$ L^{-1} = **1.29 mL $\cdot$ kg^{-1} $\cdot$ min^{-1}**

4. *Calculate the METs from a client exercising at 34.1 mL $\cdot$ kg^{-1} $\cdot$ min^{-1}.*
   a. 34.1 mL $\cdot$ kg^{-1} $\cdot$ min^{-1} $\div$ 3.5 (mL $\cdot$ kg^{-1} $\cdot$ min^{-1})/MET = **9.7 METs**

5. *Calculate the relative $\dot{V}O_2$ of a client exercising at 6.5 METs.*
   a. 6.5 METs $\times$ 3.5 (mL $\cdot$ kg^{-1} $\cdot$ min^{-1})/MET = **22.8 mL $\cdot$ kg^{-1} $\cdot$ min^{-1}**

6. *Calculate the absolute $\dot{V}O_2$ of a 43.9-kg client exercising at 25.1 mL $\cdot$ kg^{-1} $\cdot$ min^{-1}.*
   a. 43.0 kg $\times$ 25.1 mL $\cdot$ kg^{-1} $\cdot$ min^{-1} = 1079 mL $\cdot$ min^{-1}
   b. 1079 mL $\cdot$ min^{-1} $\times$ 0.001 L $\cdot$ mL^{-1} = **1.08 L $\cdot$ min^{-1}**

7. *Calculate the energy expenditure (kcal $\cdot$ min^{-1}) of a client exercising at a $\dot{V}O_2$ of 3.6 mL $\cdot$ kg^{-1} $\cdot$ min^{-1}.*
   a. 3.6 L $\cdot$ min^{-1} $\times$ 5 kcal $\cdot$ L^{-1} = **17.5 kcal $\cdot$ min^{-1}**

8. *Calculate the absolute $\dot{V}O_2$ of a client exercising at 7.3 kcal $\cdot$ min^{-1}.*
   a. 7.3 kcal $\cdot$ min^{-1} $\times$ 5 kcal $\cdot$ L^{-1} = **1.46 L $\cdot$ min^{-1}**

9. *Calculate the total energy expenditure (kcal) of a client who exercised for 25 min at 11.2 kcal $\cdot$ min^{-1}.*
   a. 25 min $\times$ 11.2 kcal $\cdot$ min^{-1} = **280 kcal**

10. *Calculate the length of the session of a client who exercised at a rate of 5.4 kcal $\cdot$ min^{-1} and expended 245 kcal.*
    a. 245 kcal $\div$ 5.4 kcal $\cdot$ min^{-1} = **45.4 min**

11. *Calculate the fat loss (lb) of a client over a 2-week period who expended an extra 544 kcal each of 7 days through exercise. Assume there was no change in diet intake.*
    a. 544 kcal $\cdot$ day^{-1} $\times$ 2 weeks $\times$ 7 day $\cdot$ week^{-1} = 7616 kcal
    b. 7616 kcal $\div$ 3500 kcal $\cdot$ lb^{-1} = **2.2 lb**

12. *Calculate the length of time required for a client to lose 5 lb who has increased her daily exercise by 500 kcal and decreased her dietary intake by 300 kcal.*
   a. 5 lb × 3500 kcal · lb^{-1} = 17,500 kcal (total energy deficit needed)
   b. 500 kcal · day^{-1} + 300 kcal · day^{-1} = 800 kcal · day^{-1} (total daily energy deficit)
   c. 17,500 kcal ÷ 800 kcal · day^{-1} = **22 days**

13. *Calculate the relative $\dot{V}O_2$ from walking on a treadmill at 3.3 mph with a 4% grade.*
   a. 3.3 mph × 26.8 (m · min^{-1})/mph = 88.4 m · min^{-1}
   b. [0.1 × 88.4 m · min^{-1}] + [1.8 × 88.4 m · min^{-1} × 0.04] + 3.5 mL · kg^{-1} · min^{-1} = **18.7 mL · kg^{-1} · min^{-1}**

14. *Calculate the relative $\dot{V}O_2$ of a 124-lb female who used a Monark leg ergometer at 70 rpm with 1.5 kg of resistance.*
   a. 124 lb ÷ 2.2 kg · lb^{-1} = 56.4 kg
   b. (70 rpm × 6 m · rev^{-1}) × 1.5 kg = 630 kg-m · min^{-1}
   c. 630 kg-m · min^{-1} ÷ 6 (kg-m · min^{-1})/W = 105 W
   d. [10.8 × 105 W ÷ 56.4 kg] + 3.5 mL · kg^{-1} · min^{-1} = **23.6 mL · kg^{-1} · min^{-1}**

15. *Calculate the relative $\dot{V}O_2$ of a 196-lb male stepping on a 9 in. bench at 30 steps · min^{-1}.*
   a. 196 lb ÷ 2.2 kg · lb^{-1} = 89.1 kg
   b. 9 in × 0.0254 m · in^{-1} = 0.229 m
   c. [0.2 × 30 steps · min^{-1}] + [1.33 × 1.8 × 30 steps · min^{-1} × 0.229 m] + 3.5 mL · kg^{-1} · min^{-1} = **40.3 mL · kg^{-1} · min^{-1}**

16. *A 122-lb female is running on a treadmill at 7.8 mph at 2% grade for 30 min. Estimate the*
   a. *relative $\dot{V}O_2$*
      i. 7.8 mph × 26.8 (m · min^{-1})/mph = 209.0 m · min^{-1}
      ii. [0.2 × 209.0 m · min^{-1}] + [0.9 × 209.0 m · min^{-1} × 0.02] + 3.5 mL · kg^{-1} · min^{-1} = **49.1 mL · kg^{-1} · min^{-1}**
   b. *METs*
      i. 49.1 mL · kg^{-1} · min^{-1} ÷ 3.5 MET/(mL · kg^{-1} · min^{-1}) = **14.0 METs**
   c. *total energy expenditure (kcal)*
      i. 122 lb ÷ 2.2 kg · lb^{-1} = 55.5 kg
      ii. 49.1 mL · kg^{-1} · min^{-1} × 55.5 kg = 2725 mL · min^{-1}
      iii. 2725 mL · min^{-1} ÷ 1000 mL · L^{-1} = 2.73 L · min^{-1}
      iv. 2.73 L · min^{-1} × 5 kcal · min^{-1}/(L · min^{-1}) = 13.65 kcal · min^{-1}
      v. 13.65 kcal · min^{-1} × 30 min = **410 kcal**

17. *A 52-kg client is cycling at 60 rpm on a Monark ergometer with a force of 1.5 kp. Determine how many 30-min sessions of this he would need to perform in order to lose 8 lb of fat.*
   a. 1.5 kp = 1.5 kg
   b. (60 rpm × 6 m · rev^{-1}) × 1.5 kg = 540 kg-m · min^{-1}
   c. 540 kg-m · min^{-1} ÷ 6 (kg-m · min^{-1})/W = 90 W
   d. [10.8 × 90 W / 52 kg] + 3.5 mL · kg^{-1} · min^{-1} = 22.2 mL · kg^{-1} · min^{-1}
   e. 22.2 mL · kg^{-1} · min^{-1} × 52 kg = 1154 mL · min^{-1}
   f. 1154 mL · min^{-1} × 0.001 L · mL^{-1} = 1.54 L · min^{-1}
   g. 1.54 L · min^{-1} × 5 kcal · L^{-1} = 7.7 kcal · min^{-1}
   h. 7.7 kcal · min^{-1} × 30 min · session^{-1} = 231 kcal · session^{-1}
   i. 8 lb × 3500 kcal · lb^{-1} = 28,000 kcal (total energy deficit needed)
   j. 28,000 kcal ÷ 231 kcal · session^{-1} = **121 sessions**

18. *A 181-lb woman is walking on a treadmill at 2.2 mph at a 5% grade. Calculate her*
   a. *gross absolute $\dot{V}O_2$*
      i. 181 lb × 2.2 kg · lb^{-1} = 82.3 kg
      ii. 2.2 mph × 26.8 (m · min^{-1})/mph = 59.0 m · min^{-1}
      iii. [0.1 × 59.0 m · min^{-1}] + [1.8 × 59.0 m · min^{-1} × 0.05] + 3.5 mL · kg^{-1} · min^{-1} = 14.7 mL · kg^{-1} · min^{-1}
      iv. 14.7 mL · kg^{-1} · min^{-1} × 82.3 kg = 1210 mL · min^{-1}
      v. 1210 mL · min^{-1} × 0.001 L · mL^{-1} = **1.21 L · min^{-1}**
   b. *net relative $\dot{V}O_2$*
      vi. 14.7 mL · kg^{-1} · min^{-1} - 3.5 mL · kg^{-1} · min^{-1} = **11.2 mL · kg^{-1} · min^{-1}**
   c. *energy expenditure in kcal · min^{-1}*
      vii. 1.21 L · min^{-1} × 5 kcal · L^{-1}) = **6.1 kcal · min^{-1}**

19. *Calculate the stepping rate on a 6-in. step of 72-kg client who you wish to exercise at 5 METs.*
   a. 5 METs × 3.5 (mL · kg^{-1} · min^{-1})/MET = 17.5 mL · kg^{-1} · min^{-1}
   b. 5 in × 0.0254 m · in^{-1} = 0.127 m
   c. [stepping equation]: 17.5 mL · kg^{-1} · min^{-1} = [0.2 × Stepping rate (steps · min^{-1})] + [1.33 × 1.8 × Stepping rate (steps · min^{-1}) × 0.127 m] + 3.5 mL · kg^{-1} · min^{-1}
   d. [steps to separate unknown]:
      i. 17.5 mL · kg^{-1} · min^{-1} - 3.5 mL · kg^{-1} · min^{-1} = [0.2 × Stepping rate (steps · min^{-1})] + [1.33 × 1.8 × Stepping rate (steps · min^{-1}) × 0.127 m]
      ii. 17.5 mL · kg^{-1} · min^{-1} - 3.5 mL · kg^{-1} · min^{-1} = Stepping rate (steps · min^{-1}) × [(0.2) + (1.33 × 1.8 × 0.127)]
      iii. [17.5 mL · kg^{-1} · min^{-1} - 3.5 mL · kg^{-1} · min^{-1}] ÷ [(0.2) + (1.33 × 1.8 × 0.127)] = Stepping rate (steps · min^{-1}) = **28 steps · min^{-1}**

20. *A 151-lb client wants to lose 15 lb of fat over the next 26 weeks. Assuming she will not change her dietary intake, calculate how long would each daily run need to be if she runs at 5.0 mph on a level treadmill.*
   a. 151 lb ÷ 2.2 kg · min^{-1} = 68.6 kg
   b. 5.0 mph × 26.8 (m · min^{-1})/mph = 134.0 m · min^{-1}
   c. [0.2 × 34.0 m^1 · min^{-1}] + [0.9 × 59.0 m · min^{-1} × 0.00] + 3.5 mL · kg^{-1} · min^{-1} = 30.3 mL · kg^{-1} · min^{-1}
   d. 30.3 mL · kg^{-1} · min^{-1} × 68.6 kg = 1836 mL · min^{-1}
   e. 1836 mL · min^{-1} × 0.001 L · mL^{-1} = 1.84 L · min^{-1}
   f. 1.84 L · min^{-1} × 5 kcal · min^{-1} /(L · min^{-1}) = 9.2 kcal · min^{-1}
   g. 26 weeks × 7 day · week^{-1} = 168 days = 168 sessions
   h. 15 lb × 3500 kcal · lb^{-1} = 52,500 kcal (total energy deficit needed)
   i. 52,500 kcal ÷ 168 sessions = 313 kcal · session^{-1}
   j. 313 kcal · session^{-1} ÷ 9.2 (kcal · min^{-1})/session = **34 min**

21. *Calculate the resistance on a Monark leg-cycle ergometer needed for a 230-lb client to cycle at 50 rpm and an intensity of 6 METs.*
   a. 230 lb ÷ 2.2 kg · lb^{-1} = 104.5 kg
   b. 6 METs × 3.5 (mL · kg^{-1} · min^{-1})/MET = 21.0 mL · kg^{-1} · min^{-1}
   c. [original leg cycling equation]: 21.0 mL · kg^{-1} · min^{-1} = [10.8 × Power (W) ÷ 104.5 kg] + 3.5 mL · kg^{-1} · min^{-1}
   d. [steps to separate unknown]
      i. 21.0 mL · kg^{-1} · min^{-1} - 3.5 mL · kg^{-1} · min^{-1} = [10.8 × Power (W) ÷ 104.5 kg]
      ii. [21.0 mL · kg^{-1} · min^{-1} - 3.5 mL · kg^{-1} · min^{-1}] × 104.5 kg = [10.8 × Power (W)]

iii. [21.0 mL · kg⁻¹ · min⁻¹ - 3.5 mL · kg⁻¹ · min⁻¹] × 104.5 kg ÷ 10.8 =
Power (W) = 169 W

   e. 169 W ÷ 6 (kg-m· min⁻¹)/W= 1014 kg-m · min⁻¹
   f. flywheel circumference = 6 m
   g. 50 rpm × 6 m · rev⁻¹ = 300 m · min⁻¹
   h. 1014 kg-m · min⁻¹ ÷ 300 m · min⁻¹ = **3.4 kg**

22. *Predict the number of weeks required for a 185-lb male to lose 20 lb of fat who will run for 45 min at a V̇O₂ of 37.5 mL·kg⁻¹·min⁻¹ three times weekly. Assume no change in his dietary intake.*

   a. 185 lb ÷ 2.2 kg · lb⁻¹ = 84.1 kg
   b. 37.5 mL · kg⁻¹ · min⁻¹ × 84.1 kg = 3154 mL · min⁻¹
   c. 3154 mL · min⁻¹ × 0.001 L · mL⁻¹ = 3.15 L · min⁻¹
   d. 3.15 L · min⁻¹ × 5 kcal · L⁻¹ = 15.8 kcal · min⁻¹
   e. 15.8 kcal · min⁻¹ × 45 min · session⁻¹ × 3 sessions · week⁻¹ = 2133 kcal · week⁻¹
   f. 20 lb × kcal · lb⁻¹ = 70,000 kcal (total energy deficit needed)
   g. 70,000 kcal ÷ 2133 kcal · week⁻¹ = **33 weeks**

Physical Activity Readiness Questionnaire (PAR-Q)

Note: The information you provide in response to this survey will be kept confidential. If you are not eligible to participate or choose not to participate in the study, your responses to the health screening will be shredded to protect your privacy.

For most people, physical activity should not pose any problem or health hazard. The questionnaire has been designed to identify the small number of adults for whom physical activity may be inappropriate or those who should seek medical advice concerning the type of activity most suitable for them.

Please read the following questions and check YES or NO in response to the question as it applies to you.

Yes_____ No_____ Has a doctor said that you have a heart condition and recommended only medical supervised physical activity?

Yes_____ No_____ Do you have chest pain brought on by physical activity?

Yes_____ No_____ Have you developed chest pain in the past month?

Yes_____ No_____ Do you tend to lose consciousness or fall over as a result of dizziness?

Yes_____ No_____ Do you have a bone or joint problem that could be aggravated by the proposed physical activity?

Yes_____ No_____ Has a doctor ever recommend medication for your blood pressure or heart condition?

Yes_____ No_____ Do you have a breathing condition that is worsened by physical activity?

Yes_____ No_____ Do you have chronic or reoccurring episodes of lower back pain?

Yes_____ No_____ Do you have diabetes?

Yes_____ No_____ Do you smoke cigarettes? If so, how many packs per day?

Yes_____ No_____ Are you aware, through you own experience or a doctor's advice, of any physical reason against your exercising without medical supervision?

Yes_____ No_____ Are you taking any prescription drugs? If so, please list them here and indicate why you are taking them:

_____

_____

Is there any other health-related information you would like to share with the investigator?

Walking and Jogging Protocols to Estimate $\dot{V}O_{2max}$

1. Weigh subject weight to the nearest 0.1 kg.

2. Subject should jog 1 mile—not 1600 m—on a level surface and at a steady pace. **Do NOT allow the subject to speed up near the end of the run**. Males should not run faster than 8:00 or females faster than 9:00.

3. Immediately on finishing, record subject's HR and finishing time. Convert the finishing time to minutes and fraction of a minute.

4. Use the appropriate equation to estimate $\dot{V}O_{2max}$.

Estimation of $\dot{V}O_{2max}$ from 1-mile jog (George et al. *MSSE* 25:401-406, 1993)

$$\dot{V}O_{2max} \ (mL \cdot kg^{-1} \cdot min^{-1}) = $$
$$100.5 + [8.344 \ 3 \ sex \ (female=0, male=1)] -$$
$$[0.1636 \times weight \ (kg)] - [1.438 \times time \ (min)] - [0.1928 \times HR \ (bpm)]$$

Estimation of $\dot{V}O_{2max}$ from 1-mile walk (Kline et al. *MSSE* 19:253-259, 1987)

$$\dot{V}O_{2max} \ (mL \cdot kg^{-1} \cdot min^{-1}) = 132.853 - [0.0769 \times weight \ (kg)] -$$
$$[0.3877 \times age \ (yr)] + [6.3150 \times sex \ (female=0, male=1)] -$$
$$[3.2649 \times time \ (min)] - [0.1565 \times HR \ (bpm)]$$

Normative Data for Aerobic Power Tests

TABLE I-1
Normative Data for Aerobic Power Tests for 18–30 Year Olds
($mL \cdot kg^{-1} \cdot min^{-1}$).

Men	Excellent	>51
	Good	47-51
	Average	43-46
	Fair	37-42
	Poor	<37
Women	Excellent	>45
	Good	37-45
	Average	33-37
	Fair	29-32
	Poor	<29

Standardized Steps in Blood Pressure Measurement

1. Select an appropriately sized cuff. Bladder width should be at least 40% of arm circumference; bladder length should be at least 80% of arm circumference.

2. Locate the brachial artery along the inner upper arm (between biceps and triceps muscles) by palpation (feeling with the fingers).

3. Wrap the cuff smoothly and snugly around the arm, centering the bladder over the brachial artery. The lower margin of the cuff should be 2.5 cm (about 1 inch) above the antecubital space (the bend in the elbow). (Find the center of the bladder by folding it in half. Don't rely on cuff markings.)

4. Locate the brachial pulse by palpating on the medial aspect of the anterior surface of the elbow. Determine the level for maximal inflation by observing the pressure at which the brachial pulse (or you may use the radial pulse) is no longer palpable as the cuff is rapidly inflated and by adding 30 mm Hg. Rapidly and completely deflate the cuff. Then wait 15-30 s before reinflating.

5. Position the stethoscope over the palpated brachial artery below the cuff at the antecubital space. Earpieces should point forward. Apply the diaphragm of the stethoscope with light pressure, ensuring skin contact at all points.

6. Rapidly and steadily, inflate the cuff to the maximal inflation level as determined in *Step 4*. Release the air in the cuff so that the pressure falls at a rate of 2 to 3 mm Hg per second.

7. Note the systolic pressure at the onset of at least two consecutive beats (*Phase* 1 Korotkoff sound). Blood pressure levels should always be recorded in even numbers and read to the nearest 2 mm Hg mark on the manometer.

8. Continue deflating the cuff and note the diastolic pressure at muffling (*Phase* 4 sound for children) and cessation of sound (*Phase* 5 sound) for adults. Listen for 10 to 20 mm Hg below the last sound heard to confirm disappearance, and then deflate the cuff rapidly and completely.

9. Record SPB and DBP. When the pressure at *Phase* 4 is recorded, the pressure at *Phase* 5 should also be recorded. Example: 120/80/74. Also, record the person's position, cuff size, and the arm used for the measurement. Typically, though, only Phase 1 and 5 sounds are used.

10. Wait 1-2 min before repeating the pressure measurement in the same arm to permit the release of blood trapped in the arm veins.

APPENDIX K

Measuring Blood Lactate Concentration and Hematocrit

Note: You should be properly trained by your instructor beforehand on how to safely sample blood. Furthermore, you are required to wear latex gloves any time you sample or analyze blood!

DRAWING BLOOD FROM A FINGER STICK

1. If blood lactate concentration is to be measured, check with the instructor to see if the lactate analyzer has been properly warmed up and calibrated.

2. Set out everything that will, or could, be needed before getting ready to draw blood. This includes at least: 2-3 alcohol swabs, several gauze pads, 2-3 lancet needles, 3-4 heparinized capillary tubes, and the autolancet fitted with a clean needle and platform. Leave the needle cap in place until just before lancing the subject. Have all materials placed so that they can be reached easily and quickly!

3. Keep in mind that many subjects are uncomfortable being stuck, so instill confidence in them by knowing—or at least acting like you know—what you are doing. When the time arrives to draw blood, do so quickly and efficiently.

4. Position the subject's hand with the palm-side up on something stable (e.g., the front safety bar of the treadmill). Select either the fourth or fifth fingertip as these are likely to have fewer calluses and thinner skin on them.

5. Vigorously scrub the area with an alcohol swab. Allow the area to dry completely before lancing the finger. After disinfecting, don't contaminate the area by touching it. If this occurs, clean the area again.

6. Twist off cap to the needle. While holding the subject's finger with one hand, firmly place the autolancet with the other hand against the fingertip and press the release button. Do not squeeze the finger yet. Place the autolancet aside. Note: Lancing slightly to the side of the fingertip will likely be less painful to the subject as there tend to be fewer nerve endings. Moreover, there is probably less callus buildup and will allow for a better sampling of blood.

7. Grab a gauze pad, gently squeeze the fingertip and wipe off the first drops of blood.

8. Again, gently squeeze the fingertip and place an end of the capillary tube in the blood droplets at a downward angle to the fingertip—blood will be pulled up the tube through capillary action.

9. After capillary tube is nearly filled, set aside and press a gauze pad on puncture site. Instruct subject to hold in place. Should subject begin feeling dizzy or lightheaded, immediately sit subject down on the floor and have him/her lean forward with the head over the legs.

10. Place the needle, gauze pads, and anything else that touched blood into a sharps biohazard container!

BLOOD DRAWING TIPS

1. Avoid lifting the capillary tube out of the blood; otherwise, air bubbles will be introduced into the tube.

2. If a bubble is introduced, it can sometimes be eliminated by holding the capillary tube in a vertical position and letting the blood drain out until the bubble is eliminated.

3. If numerous bubbles have been drawn up, discard the tube and begin over with a new capillary tube.

4. If the blood flow is not sufficient, try "milking" the finger and forcing more blood out of the puncture. However, avoid hard squeezing as this can result in altered lactate concentrations.

5. There will be times when the blood flow is inadequate despite efforts of milking the finger. In these instances, quickly re-clean the site and lance the finger again.

SAMPLING BLOOD FOR HEMATOCRIT (HCT) DETERMINATION (EXPRESSED AS A PERCENTAGE OF BLOOD CELLS TO TOTAL BLOOD VOLUME)

1. All Hcts should be sampled in duplicate.

2. Plug one end of the capillary tube by quickly sticking one end of the tube <u>perpendicular</u> into the clay.

3. Place each capillary tube into the hematocrit centrifuge with the plugged end pointing outward. Screw the flat lid over the tubes before closing the centrifuge lid. *Don't forget this step!*

4. Centrifuge the capillary tubes for 5 min at about 1800 rpm.

5. Place a capillary tube in the hematocrit reader with the plugged end pointing inward. Position the tube so that the top of the clay plug is on the "0%" line of the reader; turn the dial until the 100% line is positioned at the bottom of the meniscus of the top of the plasma.

6. Read the Hct as at the line that intersects the division between the packed blood cells and plasma.

Skinfold Measurements

The development of skinfold (anthropometric) measurements came as the result of investigations for simpler and less expensive methods of estimating body composition. Body circumferences and/or skinfold thickness are used in a regression equation, of which there are many available, for prediction of body composition. Among the most commonly employed are the Jackson and Pollock generalized equations for use with skinfold measurements developed for adult males[18] and females[19]. They are termed generalized because they are most accurate in predicting body composition of people with average amounts of body fat. Generalized equations tend to be less accurate with the very lean (e.g. athletes), obese, young, old, or other special populations. Other, more appropriate, equations have been developed for such populations, which increase their accuracy for prediction of body composition.

The major source of error in anthropometry lies in the actual skinfold measurement. Making accurate skinfold measurements is more than simply pinching the skin somewhere around a particular area and measuring the thickness. There are precise sites on which the measurements are to be taken. A well-trained technician can obtain results that approach the precision of underwater weighing. Unfortunately, most people who take skinfold measurements are not well trained. Obtaining consistently accurate skinfold measurements requires training and experience.

To take a skinfold measurement, first determine the correct measurement site. Grab the skin with the thumb and forefinger about 0.5 in. (1-2 cm) from the measurement site following the natural fold of the skin. Lift the skin up from the muscle, apply the calipers, and wait for 4 s before reading the calipers. Fat is compressible, so reading the scale before or after the 4-s delay may affect the results.

MEASUREMENT SITES

Triceps Skinfold

Along the midline on the back of the triceps of the right arm, determine the midpoint located between the top of the acromial process (top of the shoulder) to the bottom of the olecranon process of the ulna (elbow). Pinch the skin so that the fold is running vertically.

Pectoral (Chest) Skinfold

Using a line from the fold of the axillary (armpit) to the nipple, determine the midpoint (Figure L.2). Pinch the skin with the fold running in the same direction of the line.

Abdominal Skinfold

Select a site on the right side about 1 in. (2.5 cm) lateral from and 0.5 in. (1-2 cm) below the umbilicus (bellybutton) (Figure L.3). Lift a horizontal fold of skin for the measurement. NOTE: The Jackson and Pollock (1978) and Jackson and Pollock (1985) abdominal skinfolds were made using a vertical fold. Consequently, one should stay consistent with how the original equations were validated when using these equations.

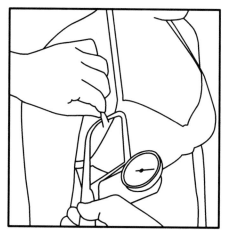

FIGURE L.2. Chest

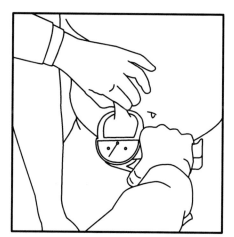

FIGURE L.3. Abdomen

Suprailiac Skinfold

Determine the midaxillary line and palpate for the iliac crest (top of the hip bone) (Figure L.4). Grasp the skin that follows the natural fold, which will follow a line of approximately from the suprailiac to the umbilicus (bellybutton), an angle of approximately 30°.

Thigh Skinfold

Determine the midline of the front of the thigh and measure midway between the inguinal crease (the natural crease between the thigh and hip which is at an approximate 45°) and the top of the patella (kneecap) (Figure L.5). Grasp a vertical fold of skin for the measurement.

ESTIMATION OF BODY DENSITY

There are two calculation steps for determining percent fat: determining body density and then using body density to estimate percent fat. All the skinfold

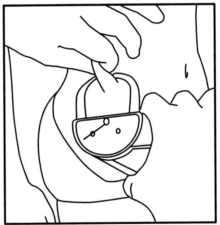

FIGURE L.4. Iliac

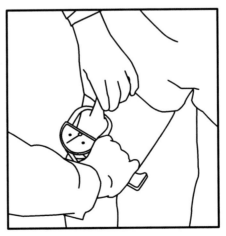

FIGURE L.5. Thigh

TABLE L.1

Formulas for calculating body density from Jackson and Pollock skinfold equations.

Females:	Body Density = 1.0994921 - 0.0009929 × sum + 0.0000023 × sum² - 0.0001392 × age
	(triceps, suprailiac, thigh skinfold measurements)
Males:	Body Density = 1.1093800 - 0.0008267 × sum + 0.0000016 × sum² - 0.0002574 × age
	(chest, abdominal, thigh skinfold measurements)

equations estimate body density from the measurements, which is then used to estimate percent fat. Two generalized equations that have withstood the test of numerous cross-validation studies are ones published by Jackson and Pollock for men[18] and women[19]. Each study developed numerous equations based on different skinfold measurements, although they all were similar in prediction error. Listed below are a single equation from each study based on the sum of three skinfold measurements. Standard errors of their formulae ranged from 3.6% to 3.8%. The potential errors are increased if these equations are used on the young or old, very lean and muscular or obese. Other population specific equations are available and more suitable for these groups.

ESTIMATION OF PERCENT FAT

The two most commonly used equations for estimating percent fat from body density are the Siri[35] and Brozek[3] formulas. A limitation to these formulas is that they assume the density of fat-free mass to remain a constant across the population when in fact it varies. Thus, the actual percent fat tends to be slightly higher than the measured percent fat in the lean, muscular individual and the opposite in obese individuals.

TABLE L.2

Siri and Brozek formulas for conversion of body density to percent body fat.

Siri	Percent Fat = [(495 / Body Density) -450] × 100
Brozek	Percent Fat = [(4.570 / Body Density) - 4.142] × 100

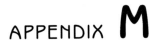

Normative Data for Body Composition

TABLE M.1
Normative Data for Body Composition for 18–30 Year Olds

Men	Excellent	≤7%
	Good	8-12%
	Average	13-16%
	Fair	17-19%
	Poor	>20%
Women	Excellent	<14%
	Good	15-19%
	Average	20-24%
	Fair	25-29%
	Poor	>30%

Determining Ideal Body Weight

If the percent fat is above the ideal range for percent fat, use this table to calculate the amount of weight loss required in order to achieve the ideal percent fat. This calculation assumes that all of the weight loss is from fat.

1. *Determine the amount of fat-free weight*
   a. Multiply the current weight by the fraction of the current percent fat. This calculates the amount of fat weight.
   b. Subtract the fat weight from the current weight to obtain the fat-free weight.

2. *Determine the ideal body weight*
   a. Divide the fat-free weight by the percent of the ideal fat-free weight (e.g. if the ideal percent fat is 15%, then the fraction of the ideal fat-free weight is (1 – 0.15) or 0.85).

   <u>Example</u>. If the current weight is 75 kg and percent fat is 20%, and goal is to achieve 15%, then:

1. *Determine the amount of fat-free weight*
   fat weight: 75 kg × 0.20 = 15 kg
   fat-free weight: 75 kg – 15 kg = 60 kg

2. *Determine the ideal body weight*
   60 kg / (1 – 0.15) = 70.6 kg

STPD Correction Factors

TABLE O-1
Correction factors of moist gas to STPD.

Barometric Pressure (mm Hg)	Temperature (°C)														
	18	19	20	21	22	23	24	25	26	27	28	29	30	31	32
700	0.842	0.838	0.834	0.829	0.825	0.821	0.816	0.812	0.807	0.802	0.797	0.793	0.788	0.783	0.778
705	0.848	0.844	0.840	0.836	0.831	0.827	0.822	0.818	0.813	0.809	0.803	0.799	0.794	0.788	0.784
710	0.855	0.850	0.846	0.842	0.837	0.833	0.828	0.824	0.819	0.814	0.809	0.804	0.799	0.795	0.790
715	0.861	0.857	0.854	0.840	0.843	0.839	0.834	0.830	0.825	0.821	0.815	0.811	0.806	0.801	0.796
720	0.867	0.863	0.858	0.854	0.849	0.845	0.840	0.836	0.831	0.826	0.821	0.816	0.812	0.807	0.802
725	0.873	0.869	0.865	0.860	0.855	0.851	0.846	0.842	0.837	0.832	0.828	0.823	0.817	0.812	0.807
730	0.879	0.875	0.871	0.866	0.861	0.857	0.852	0.847	0.843	0.838	0.833	0.828	0.823	0.818	0.813
735	0.886	0.881	0.877	0.872	0.868	0.863	0.858	0.854	0.849	0.844	0.839	0.834	0.829	0.824	0.819
740	0.892	0.887	0.883	0.878	0.874	0.869	0.864	0.860	0.855	0.850	0.845	0.840	0.835	0.830	0.825
745	0.898	0.894	0.889	0.885	0.880	0.875	0.871	0.866	0.861	0.856	0.851	0.846	0.841	0.836	0.831
750	0.904	0.900	0.895	0.890	0.886	0.881	0.876	0.872	0.867	0.862	0.857	0.852	0.847	0.842	0.837
755	0.910	0.908	0.901	0.897	0.892	0.887	0.882	0.878	0.873	0.868	0.863	0.858	0.853	0.848	0.843
760	0.916	0.912	0.907	0.902	0.898	0.893	0.888	0.883	0.879	0.874	0.869	0.864	0.859	0.854	0.848
765	0.923	0.918	0.914	0.910	0.904	0.899	0.896	0.890	0.885	0.880	0.875	0.870	0.865	0.860	0.854
770	0.928	0.924	0.919	0.915	0.910	0.905	0.901	0.896	0.891	0.886	0.881	0.876	0.871	0.865	0.860
775	0.934	0.930	0.925	0.921	0.916	0.911	0.907	0.902	0.897	0.892	0.887	0.882	0.877	0.871	0.866

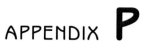

BTPS Correction Factors

TABLE P-1
Correction factor to convert a gas volume at ATPS to BTPS.

Temperature (°C)	BTPS Correction Factor
18	1.114
19	1.108
20	1.102
21	1.096
22	1.091
23	1.085
24	1.080
25	1.075
26	1.068
27	1.063
28	1.057
29	1.051
30	1.045
31	1.039
32	1.032

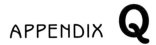

Water Density Correction Factors

TABLE Q-1
Water density at different temperatures.

Temperature (°C)	Density (g · mL^{-1})
25	0.9971
26	0.9968
27	0.9965
28	0.9963
29	0.9960
30	0.9957
31	0.9954
32	0.9951
33	0.9947
34	0.9944
35	0.9941
36	0.9937
37	0.9934
38	0.9930

GLOSSARY

Bicarbonate (HCO$_3^-$): Found primarily in blood, bicarbonate serves to buffer the acid produced during high-intensity exercise.

Blood lactate concentration: Lactate produced by muscle is transported into blood of which the blood concentration reflects the difference in lactate appearance and removal by muscle, the heart, and liver.

Cardiac output (Q̇): The rate of blood pumped from the heart, usually expressed as liters per minute.

Carnitine palmityl transferase: A mitochondrial enzyme associated with beta oxidation.

Creatine kinase (CK or CPK): The sarcoplasmic enzyme responsible for transferring a high-energy phosphate to ADP to synthesize ATP.

Diastolic blood pressure (DBP): The lowest arterial blood pressure, which occurs at the end of diastole.

Epinephrine (EPI): Also known by its British name, adrenaline, EPI is one of the two catecholamines released from the adrenal glands in response to sympathetic innervation. Generally, EPI stimulates HR and promotes vasoconstriction.

Excess post-exercise oxygen consumption (EPOC): EPOC represents oxygen used by the body after exercise that is above what is needed for rest. Initially, oxygen is used to replenish myoglobin stores and to resynthesize PCr. Later, numerous other factors contribute to the increase of V̇O$_2$ above resting levels.

Glucagon: A pancreatic hormone released into blood that serves to stimulate blood release from the liver.

Glycerol: A three-carbon molecule to which three fatty acids attach to form a triglyceride molecule. During lipolysis, glycerol is released into blood, and because it is not rapidly removed from blood, glycerol is used as marker of lipolysis.

Hematocrit (Hct): The percentage of cells by volume in blood.

Insulin: A pancreatic hormone released into the blood that promotes blood glucose uptake into muscle.

Ketone bodies: Formed in the liver and kidneys from the breakdown of fatty acid metabolism, they circulate and enter tissues, which use the ketones as fuel.

Lactate threshold: The point at which the appearance of lactate in blood becomes rapidly greater than the rate of lactate removal.

Malate dehydrogenase (MDH): A mitochondrial enzyme associated with the Krebs' cycle.

Maximal oxygen consumption (V̇O$_{2max}$): The maximal rate at which oxygen can be used by the body. A high V̇O$_{2max}$ reflects a strong cardiovascular system and is associated with endurance athletes.

Mean arterial pressure (MAP): Calculated as the diastolic blood pressure and 1/3 of the difference between the systolic and diastolic blood pressures.

Minute ventilation (V̇E): The rate of expired air ventilation usually expressed as liters per minute.

Mixed arterial-venous oxygen difference (a-v O₂ diff): The difference in oxygen content between arterial and mixed venous blood. The mixed a-v O₂ diff reflects venous blood returning from all tissues of the body, not just working muscle.

Myoglobin: An oxygen-carrying molecule similar to hemoglobin, but found in muscle. Myoglobin stores and transfers O_2 from blood to the mitochondria.

Myokinase (MK, also known as adenylate kinase): The sarcoplasmic enzyme responsible for synthesizing ATP from two ADPs.

Norepinephrine (NE): Primarily a neurotransmitter, NE is also a catecholamine released from the adrenal glands.

Oxygen consumption (V̇O₂): Also referred to as oxygen uptake and oxygen consumption. Although measured at the mouth, $\dot{V}O_2$ reflects the rate at which oxygen is being utilized by the mitochondria. Moreover, $\dot{V}O_2$ is used as an indirect measure of energy expenditure if at steady-state.

Oxygen deficit (O₂D): Occurring at the onset of exercise or with an increase in exercise intensity, O_2D is the difference between the estimated $\dot{V}O_2$ and the measured $\dot{V}O_2$. O_2D reflects ATP contributed entirely by anaerobic metabolism.

Oxygen ventilatory equivalent (V̇E/V̇O₂): The ratio of $\dot{V}E$ to $\dot{V}O_2$. The point at which $\dot{V}E/\dot{V}O_2$ begins to quickly rise is often the best marker of the ventilatory threshold.

pH: A 0 to 14 logarithmic scale of H^+ concentration that is a measure of acidity (from less than 7 to 0) or alkalinity (from above 7 to 14).

Phophorylase: The sarcoplasmic enzyme responsible for the breakdown of glycogen.

Phosphofructokinase (PFK): Found in the sarcoplasm, PFK is the primary rate-limiting enzyme of glycolysis.

Rate-Pressure product (RPP): Calculated as the product of HR and SBP, RPP reflects the work performed by the heart.

Respiratory exchange ratio (RER): Calculated as the ratio of $\dot{V}CO_2$ to $\dot{V}O_2$, RER reflects the relative contribution of carbohydrate and fat utilization by the aerobic system. An RER of 0.7 indicates that 100% of fuels oxidized by the mitochondria are fats while an RER of 1.0 indicates that all of the oxidized fuels are carbohydrates; an RER of 0.83 reflects an equal contribution of carbohydrate and fat oxidation. This ratio incorrectly assumes that no proteins are being oxidized, for which RER is also referred to as the non-protein RER.

Steady-state: An exercise metabolic rate in which the body's various physiological systems are remaining stable. Thus, parameters such as HR, $\dot{V}E$, and blood lactate concentration have increased from resting values, but are no longer rising. Because at intensities above the lactate threshold there is an upward drift for many of these parameters, steady-state refers to any intensity at or below the lactate threshold.

Stroke volume (SV): The volume of blood ejected from the heart by a single contraction.

Submaximal exercise intensity: An exercise intensity that is less than the intensity needed to elicit $\dot{V}O_{2max}$. Typically, though, submaximal intensities refer to intensities in which steady-state can be achieved.

Succinate dehydrogenase (SDH): A mitochondrial enzyme associated with the Krebs' cycle.

Supramaximal exercise intensity: An exercise intensity that is greater than the intensity needed to elicit $\dot{V}O_{2max}$.

Systolic blood pressure (SBP): The peak arterial blood pressure, which occurs at the end of systole.

Total peripheral resistance (TPR): The resistance to blood flow encountered primarily at the level of the arterioles, which can be calculated by dividing the mean arterial pressure by cardiac output. Vasoconstriction increases TPR while vasodilation decreases TPR.

Variable (dependent): The variable(s) under investigation and which is influenced by manipulations of the independent variable. For example, the investigator wishes to see what effects that air temperature (independent variable) has on core body temperature (dependent variable) and sweat rates (dependent variable) during prolonged exercise.

Variable (independent): The variable(s) controlled by the investigator. For example, the investigator controls treadmill speed (independent variable) in order to observe the effects of running speed on HR (dependent variable) and blood lactate concentration (dependent variable).

Ventilatory threshold: The point at which $\dot{V}E$ begins increasing in an exponential manner. Occurrence of the ventilatory threshold is closely associated with the lactate threshold.

REFERENCES

1. Åstrand, P-O. and K. Rodahl. *Textbook of Workbook Physiology: Physiological Bases of Exercise.* New York: McGraw-Hill Book, 1986.
2. Brooks, G.A., T.D. Fahey, T.P. White, and K.M. Baldwin. *Exercise Physiology: Human Bioenergetics and its Applications.* Boston: McGraw-Hill Higher Education, 2000.
3. Brozek, J., F. Grande, J. Anderson, et al. Densitometric analysis of body composition: revision of some quantitative assumptions. *Ann. NY Acad. Sci.* 110:113-140, 1963.
4. Brück, K. and H. Olschewski. Body temperature related factors diminishing the drive to exercise. *Can. J. Physiol. Pharm.* 65:1274-1280, 1987.
5. Coggan, A.R. and E.F. Coyle. Metabolism and performance following carbohydrate ingestion late in exercise. *Med. Sci. Sports Exerc.* 21(1):59-65, 1989.
6. Costill, D.L., G.P. Dalsky, and W.J. Fink. Effects of caffeine ingestion on metabolism and exercise performance. *Med. Sci. Sports.* 10:155-158, 1978.
7. Coyle, E.F. A.R. Coggan, M.K. Hemmert, and J.L. Ivy. Muscle glycogen utilization during prolonged strenuous exercise when fed carbohydrate. *J. Appl. Physiol.* 61(1):165-172, 1986.
8. Coyle, E.F. Cardiovascular drift during prolonged exercise and the effects of dehydration. *Int. J. Sports Med.* 19:S121-S124, 1998.
9. Febbraio, M.A., R.J. Snow, M. Hargreaves, C.G. Stathis, I.K. Martin, and M.F. Carey. Muscle metabolism during exercise and heat stress in trained men: effect of acclimation. *J. Appl. Physiol.* 76(2):589-597, 1994.
10. Fortney, S.M., E.R. Nadel, C.B. Wenger, and J.R. Bove. Effect of blood volume on sweating rate and body fluids in exercising humans. *J. Appl. Physiol. : Respirat. Environ. Exerc. Physiol.* 51(6):1594-1600, 1981.
11. Galbo, H. *Hormonal and Metabolic Adaptations to Exercise.* New York: Thieme Verlag-Stratton, 1983.
12. George, J.D., P.R. Vehrs, P.W. Allsen, G.W. Fellingham, and A.G. Fisher. VO_{2max} estimation from a submaximal 1-mile track jog for fit college-age individuals. *Med. Sci. Sports Exerc.* 25(3):401-406, 1993.
13. Hanson, P., A. Claremont, J. Dempsey, and W. Redan. *J. Appl. Physiol.: Respirat. Exerc. Environ. Physiol.* 52(3):615-623, 1982.
14. Hargreaves, M. (Ed.). *Exercise Metabolism.* Champaign, IL: Human Kinetics, 1995.
15. Hogan, M.C., R.H. Cox, and H.W. Welch. Lactate accumulation during incremental exercise with varied inspired oxygen fractions. *J. Appl. Physiol.: Respirat. Environ. Exerc. Physiol.* 55(4):1134-1140, 1983.
16. Horton, E.S. and R.L. Terjung (Eds.). *Exercise Nutrition, and Energy Metabolism.* New York: Macmillan, 1988.
17. Ivy, J.L., D.L. Costill, W.J. Fink, and R.W. Lower. Influence of caffeine and carbohydrate feedings on endurance performance. *Med. Sci. Sports.* 11:6-11, 1979.
18. Jackson, A.S. and M.L. Pollock. Generalized equations for predicting body density of men. *Br. J. Nutr.* 40:497-504, 1978.
19. Jackson, A.S. and M.L. Pollock. Practical assessment of body composition. *Physician Sportsmed.* 13:76-90, 1985.
20. Jáequier, E. Energy, obesity, and body weight standards. *Am. J. Clin Nutr* 45:1035-1047, 1987.
21. Kenney, W.L. and R.K. Anderson. Responses of older and younger women to exercise in dry and humid heat without fluid replacement. *Med. Sci. Sports Exerc.* 20(2):155-160, 1988.
22. Kline, G.M., J.P. Porcari, R. Hintermeister, P.S. Freedson, A. Ward, R.F McCarron, J. Ross, and J.M. Ripe. Estimation of VO_{2max} from a one-mile track walk, gender, age, and body weight. *Med. Sci. Sports Exerc.* 19(3):253-259, 1987.
23. Lamb, D.R. and C.V. Gisolfi (Eds.). *Perspectives in Exercise Science and Sports Medicine Volume 5: Energy Metabolism in Exercise and Sport.* Carmel, IN: Cooper, 1992.

24. McArdle, W.D., F.I. Katch, and V.L. Katch. *Exercise Physiology: Energy, Nutrition, and Human Performance.* Philadephia: Lippincott Williams & Wilkins, 2001.
25. Miller, W.C. *The Biochemistry of Exercise and Metabolic Adaptation.* Dubuque, IA: WCB Brown & Benchmark, 1992.
26. Montain, S.J. and E.F. Coyle. Influence of graded dehydration on hyperthermia and cardiovascular drift. *J. Appl. Physiol.* 73(4):1340-1350, 1992.
27. Nadel, E.R., E. Cafarelli, M.F. Roberts, and C.B Wenger. Circulatory regulation during exercise in different ambient temperatures. *J. Appl. Physiol.: Respirat. Environ. Physiol.* 46(3):430-437, 1979.
28. Owen, M.D., K.C. Kregel, P.T. Wall, and C.V. Gisolfi. Effects of ingesting carbohydrate beverages during exercise in the heat. *Med. Sci. Sports Exerc.* 18(5):568-575, 1986.
29. Pandolf, K.B., M.N. Sawka, and R.R. Gonzalez (Eds.). *Human Performance Physiology and Environmental Medicine at Terrestrial Extremes.* Indianapolis: Benchmark Press, 1988.
30. Plowman, S.A. and D.L. Smith. *Exercise Physiology for Health, Fitness, and Performance.* San Francisco: Benjamin Cummings, 2003.
31. Powers, S.K., E. Howley, and R. Cox. Ventilatory and metabolic reactions to heat stress during prolonged exercise. *J. Sports Med. Phys. Fit.* 22:32-36, 1982.
32. Powers, S.K. and E.T. Howley. *Exercise Physiology: Theory and Application to Fitness and Performance.* Dubuque, IA: Brown & Benchmark, 1997.
33. Romijin, J.A., E.F. Coyle, L.S. Sidossi, A. Gastaldelli, J.F. Horowitz, E. Endert, and R.R. Wolfe. Regulation of endogenous fat and carbohydrate metabolism in relation to exercise intensity and duration. *Am. J. Physiol. 265 (Endocrinol. Metab. 28)*:E380-E391, 1993.
34. Rowell, L.B. Human cardiovascular adjustments to exercise and thermal stress. *Physiol. Rev.* 51(1):75-159, 1974.
35. Siri, W.E. Body composition from fluid spaces and density. *Univ. Calif. Donner Lab. Med. Phys Rep.* March, 1956.
36. Terrillion, K.A., F.W. Kolkhorst, F.A. Dolgener, and S.A. Joslyn. The effect of creatine supplementation on two 700-m maximal running bouts. *Int. J. Sport Nutri.* 7(2):138-143, 1997.
37. Turcotte, L. Muscle fatty acid uptake during exercise: possible mechanisms. *Exerc. Sport Sci. Rev.* 28:4-9, 2000.
38. van Beaumont, W., J.E. Greenleaf, and L. Juhos. Disproportional changes in hematocrit, plasma volume, and proteins during exercise and bed rest. *J. Appl. Physiol.* 33(1): 55-61, 1972.
39. Wilmore, J.H. A simplified method for determination of residual lung volumes. *J. Appl. Physiol.* 27(1):96-100, 1969.
40. Wilmore, J.H. and D.L. Costill. *Physiology of Sport and Exercise.* Champaign, IL: Human Kinetics, 1999.

INDEX

Page numbers in italics followed by f denote figures; those followed by t denote tables.

Humidity, 19, 77
Hydrostatic weighing, 100

I
Ideal body weight, 98, 99, 147
Independent variables, 8
Indirect calorimetry, 42–44, *43t*
Inquiry-based research project guidelines, 121–122
International Olympic Committee (IOC), 114
Intracellular fluid (ICF), 19, 77

J
Jackson, A. S., 142, 143, 144, 145
Jackson and Pollock skinfold equations, 142, 143, 144, *145t*
Joule (J), 1, *5t, 6t*

K
Kilocalories (kcal), 43, 127
Kilograms (kg), 2, *2t*, 127–128, *128t*
Kilojoules (kj), 43
Krebs' cycle, 39, 46, 53

L
Laboratory data, working with
  components of a graph, 8, *8f*
  graph construction, 8–9, *9t*
  levels of significance and rounding, 6–7
  practice calculations, 7
  relative vs. absolute comparisons, 7–8
  statistical significance, 9–11, *9t, 10f, 11f*
  units conversation, 7
Lactate, 40, 46
  blood lactate [La], 49
  lactate production and acid buffering, 69–70, 73
  measuring blood lactate concentration and hematocrit, 140–141
Lipolysis, 114
Liter (L), 1
Liver glycogen, 61, 64

M
Margaria stair-climb test, 111
Mass (weight), 2
Maximal oxygen uptake ($\dot{V}O_{2max}$)
  developing a submaximal cycling protocol to estimate, 58–59
  direct measurement of, 53–55
  field tests for estimating, 56–57
  graded exercise and maximal aerobic power, 34

metabolic calculations and, 125–128, *125f, 126t, 128t*
  walking and jogging protocols to estimate, 137
Mean arterial blood pressure (MAP), 33
Measuring blood lactate concentration and hematocrit, 20, 140–141
Mechanical energy, 5, 39
Metabolic calculations, 125–126, *125f, 126t*
  algebraic reminders, 128–129
  converting units of power from kg-m·min^{-1} to watts, 127–128, *128t*
  kilocalorie, 127
  metabolic equivalents (METS), 126–127
  net and gross oxygen utilization, 127
Metabolic and cardiovascular expressions, rates of, 6
Metabolic problems, 130–131
  solutions to, 132–135
Metabolic responses to exercise, 39–41, *40f*
  lab activities
    direct measurement of $\dot{V}O_{2max}$, 53–55
    graded exercise, 49–52, 50t
    measuring energy expenditure, indirect calorimetry, 42–44, *43t*
  student activities
    developing a submaximal cycling protocol to estimate $\dot{V}O_{2max}$, 58–59
    field tests for estimating $\dot{V}O_{2max}$, 56–57
    oxygen deficit and EPOC, 45–48, *45f, 46f, 47f*
  virtual lab activities
    graded exercise, 67–70
    prolonged exercise, 60–62
    training effects on graded exercise, 71–73
    training effects on prolonged exercise, 63–66
Meteorological balloons, 3
Metric units, 1
  of force, *4t*
  metric equivalents of weight and mass, 2, *2t*
  metric measures of length
    conversion factors and, *2t*
    prefixes and symbols for, *1t*
  of speed (velocity), *4t*
Metropolitan Life Insurance Company, 98
Mitochondria, and ATP production, 39–40
Motoneurons, 93
Motor units, 93, 114
Muscle
  contraction of, 39
  myoglobin in, 47
Muscle glycogen, 61, 64, 92
Myocardial contractility, 13, 24, 32
Myosin heads, 39

$\dot{V}O_{2max}$. *see* Maximal oxygen uptake ($\dot{V}O_{2max}$)
Volume, 2–3

W

Walking and jogging protocols to estimate $\dot{V}O_{2max}$ 137

Water density correction factors, *150t*
Water loss, during exercise, 19–20
Watts (W), 1, *5t*, 127–128, *128t*
Weight (mass), 2. *see also* Body composition assessment
Work, power and, 3, 4, *5t*

LaVergne, TN USA
20 January 2011
213117LV00001B/15/P